JUICYLIFE
with Jenny Patrizia

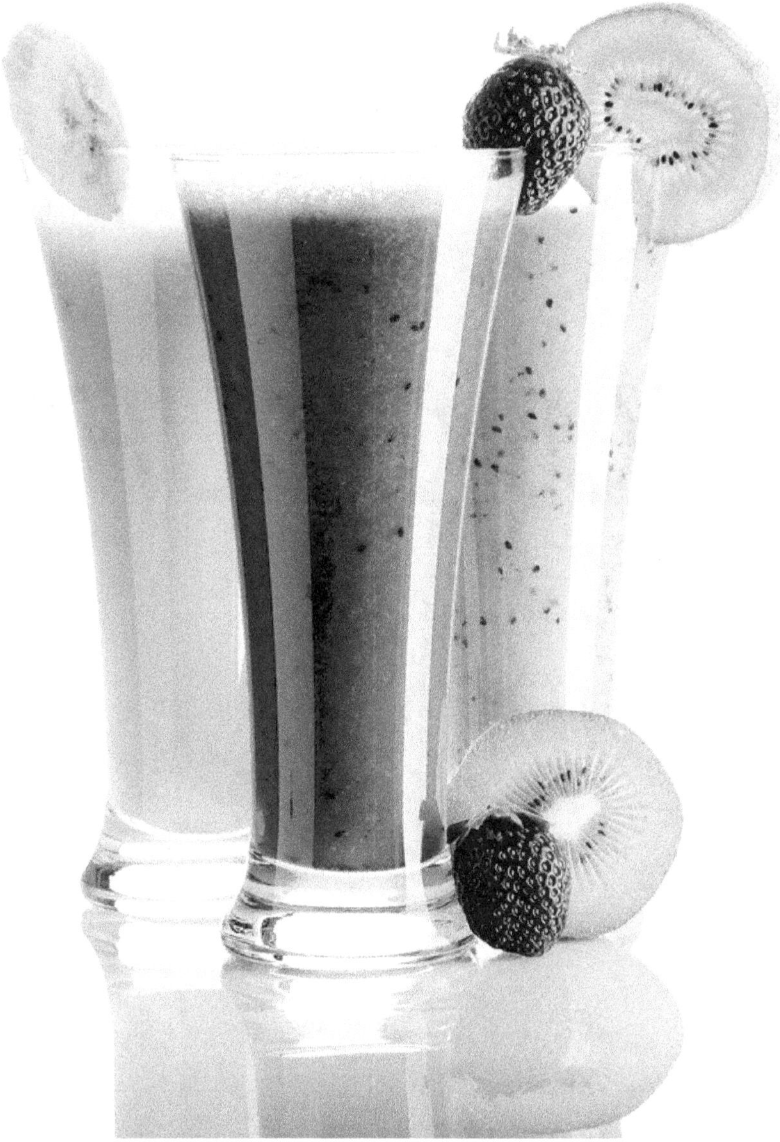

Warning: Pregnant women and moms, who are breastfeeding, should avoid lavender tea. Pregnant women, breastfeeding mothers and folks who take blood thinners should consult a doctor before consuming ginger.

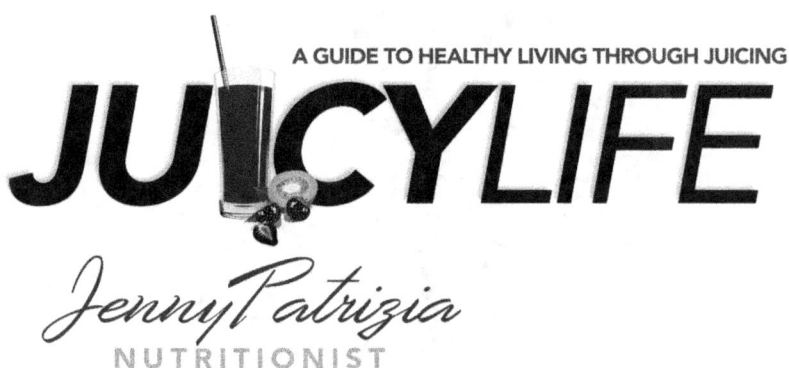

A GUIDE TO HEALTHY LIVING THROUGH JUICING

JUICYLIFE

Jenny Patrizia

NUTRITIONIST

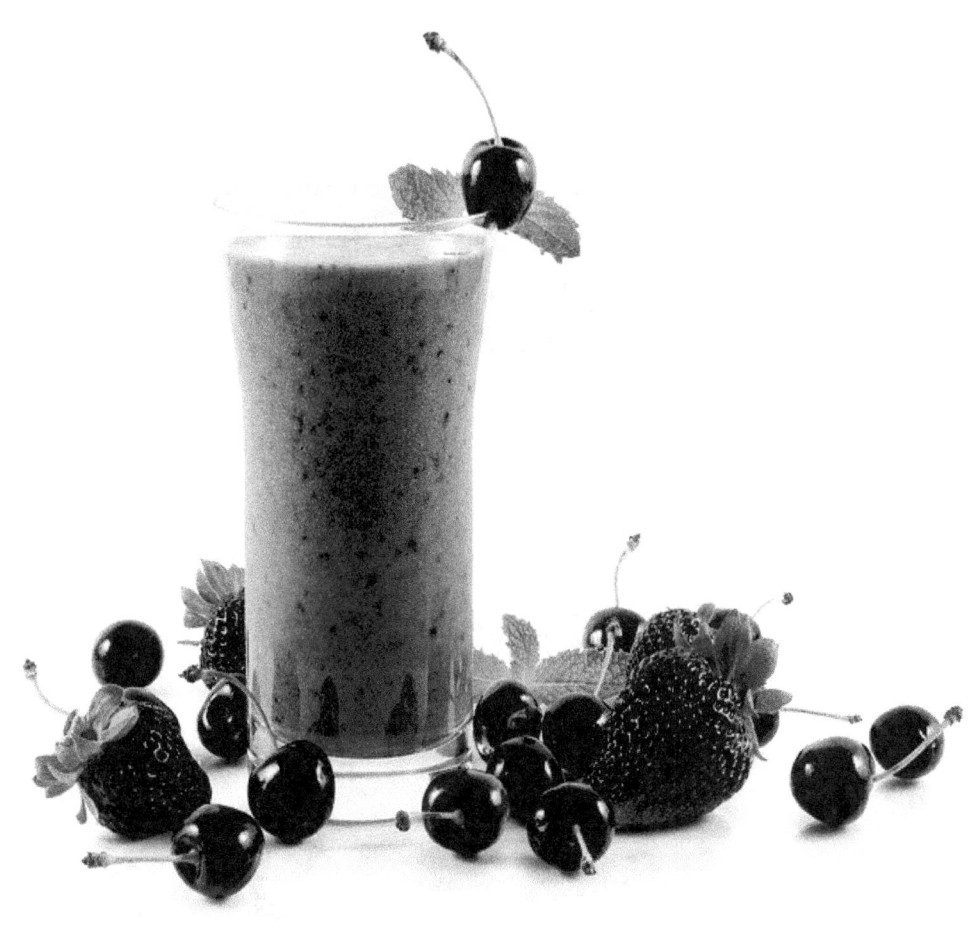

Juicy Life
Written and created by Jenny Patrizia

ISBN-13: 978-1542577823

ISBN-10: 1542577829

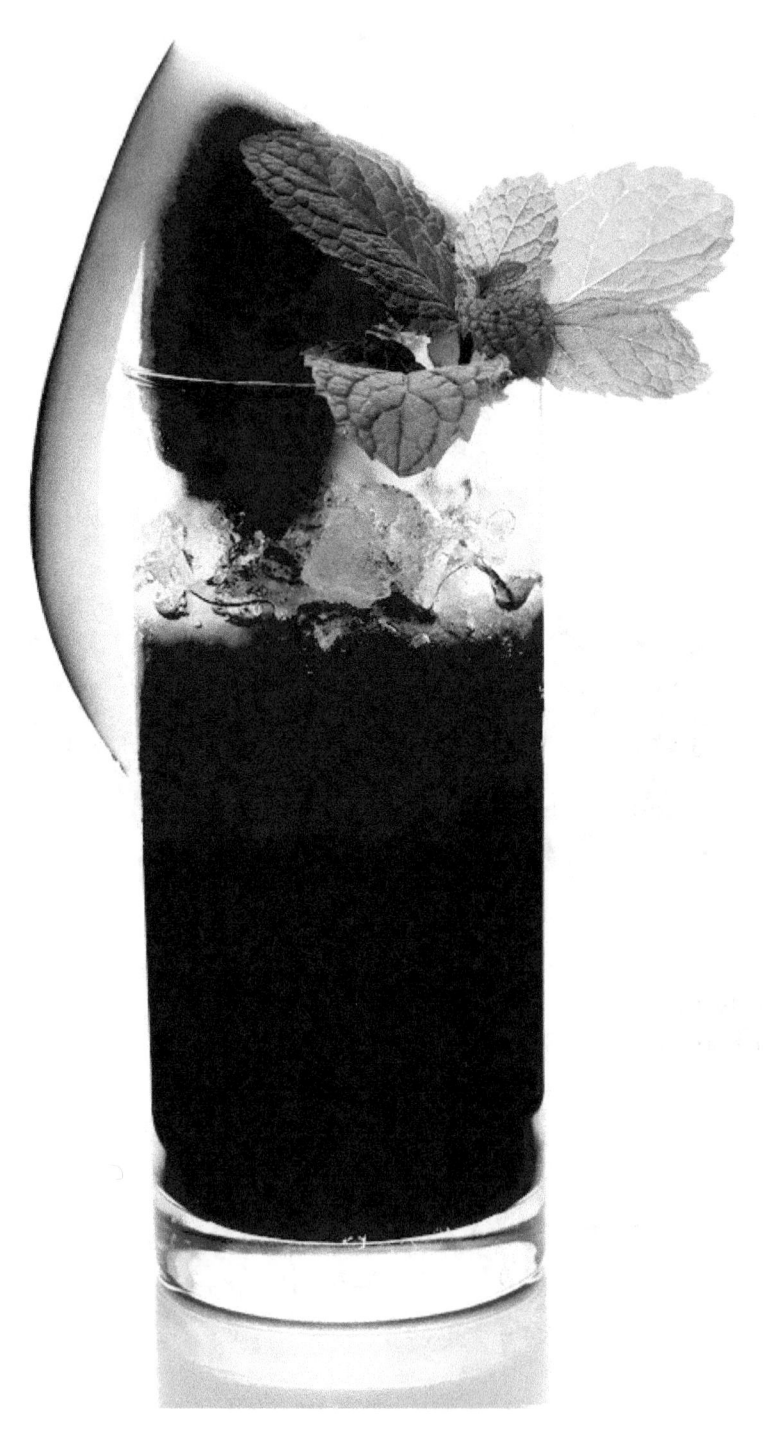

Juicy Friends,

If you are like me, trying to find ways to feed your family in the healthiest, most economical, natural way possible then The Juicy Life is for you! Whether you are a mom struggling to get your kids to eat their fruits and vegetables, or a career man or woman constantly on the go and have no time to eat healthy meals or seniors who find it challenging to chew and digest certain foods or be able to prepare nutritious meals, then the smoothie recipe book, THE JUICY LIFE, is what you have been waiting for! The Juicy Life, written and created by world known nutritionist, Jenny Patrizia, is filled with delicious fun to make juices and smoothies recipes that have the potential to help fight off certain illnesses and/or help alleviate its bothersome symptoms, naturally. Fruits and vegetables contain certain properties that can actually help reduce symptoms of certain illnesses or health concerns many of us face today.

The Juicy Life includes recipes that contain natural vitamins and minerals found in everyday fruits and vegetables whose properties can help battle insomnia, lower blood pressure, control acne breakouts, reduce anxiety & depression, help alleviate menopause, migraines, arthritis pain and menstrual cramps symptoms, decrease congestion, reduce varicose veins, wrinkles and cellulite, ease allergies and asthma, aid in weight loss and so much more! There is a customized, nutrient rich smoothie just for anyone whose looking to live a JUICY LIFE!

Smoothies/Juices are:
1. Nutritious

Smoothies provide vitamins, minerals, protein, fiber and healthy fats necessary for good nutrition. Fat is required for proper body functions and burned by your body for energy. Some of these healthy fats added to smoothies are egg yolks, coconut oil and creams.

2. Helps Keep You Hydrated

A smoothie for breakfast helps you get hydrated at the start of the day, unlike soda and coffee. Since your body pulls water from many foods in order to stay hydrated, you won't have to drink water when you're drinking juices. Did you know that milk and yogurt are largely water, so if your smoothie is dairy-based, it will keep you hydrated.

3. Provide Calcium

Smoothies made with dairy products provide calcium for bone strength. Eight ounces of milk provide almost a third of your daily requirement of calcium. Win-win situation! Add milk that is fortified with Vitamin D and you have a high nutrient beverage.

4. Simple and Fun to Make

Choose a banana, cup of berries, shredded coconut, frozen fruit, vanilla extract or other fruit and flavor combination. Fresh pineapple with shredded coconut is quite tropical; strawberries and fresh cream make a great summer treat.

5. Make a Healthy Breakfast on the Go

A homemade smoothie for your breakfast makes an easy and quick meal. A nutritious smoothie packs more nutrition than most multivitamins.

6. Economical

Smoothies help you save money as well as time. They are so easy even kids can do them (of course always under adult supervision).

7. Gives Your Body Fiber

Fiber is essential in helping clean out the body while removing toxins. Add a teaspoon of fiver to your smoothie and you are good to go.

8. Helps You Fight Flu Season

Smoothies are loaded with vitamins and minerals that increase your body's immune system.

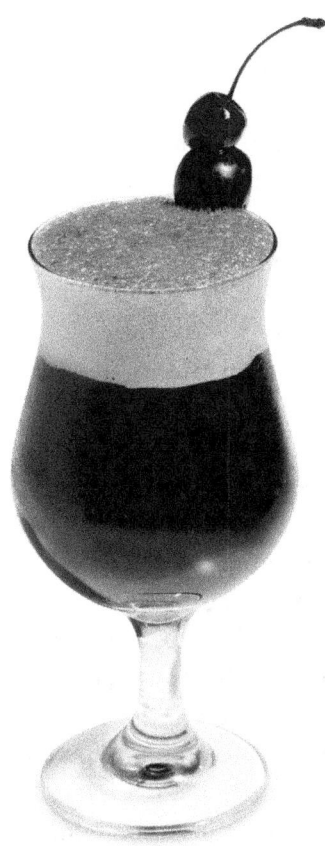

Fruits and Vegetables
Fun Facts

- Bananas are actually an herb, not a fruit. It is in fact related to the orchid and lily families. The bananas are actually considered the berries of this giant herb.
- Eating an apple is a more reliable method of staying awake than consuming a cup of coffee because the sugar in an apple is stronger than the caffeine in coffee.
- Rice has more varieties than any other fruit or vegetable. Many countries have a few specific varieties of rice that cannot be found anywhere else.
- The cabbage contains almost as much water as watermelon. Watermelon is 92% water, cabbage is 90%.
- Peanuts are not nuts; they are part of the pea family. Peanut oil can be utilized to make nitroglycerin, a major component of dynamite.
- Pumpkins are not a vegetable, they are a fruit. So are avocados.
- Almonds are not nuts, they are considered to be a member of the peach family.
- Darker green vegetables contain more vitamin C than lighter green vegetables.
- Tomatoes are not a vegetable, they are a fruit. They were once considered a type of apple by France and Italy and used to be yellow, not orange or red.
- A stalk of celery only contains 10 calories. The human body uses more calories digesting celery, and so celery is called a negative food.
- The hotter a chili pepper is, the healthier it is. This is because chili peppers contain capsaicin, which is what

gives the chili pepper its heat. Capsaicin is also utilized to treat various ailments, such as arthritis, and to help lower blood cholesterol or the risk of prostrate cancer.

- Smaller chili peppers are usually hotter than larger chili peppers. Habanera chili peppers are some of the hottest chili peppers in the world.
- Potato plants are grown from cutting up a potato into pieces and planting them in the ground. Each piece eventually grows into a separate potato plant.
- Tofu, and Miso Paste and Soy Sauce are all made from soybeans.
- Bananas are known for potassium, but potassium is actually found in good quantities in most fruits and vegetables. The avocado has more than double the amount of potassium than a banana.
- In an emergency, coconut water can be substituted for blood plasma.
- Carrots were originally red, purple, yellow or white. Orange carrots were not produced until the 16th century,
- Smaller zucchini is much more flavorful than larger zucchini.
- Refrigerated tomatoes will lose flavor and nutrients.
- Never store onions and potatoes together. They both produce gases that when in close proximity to each other, cause both of them to spoil much faster.
- When storing potatoes, placing an apple with them will help prevent the potatoes from sprouting.

Fruit Calories Chart	
Fruit and Serving Size	Calories
Apple, 1 raw apple with skin	81
Apricots, 3 medium	51
Avocado, 5oz or 145g	250
Banana, 1 medium	105
Blackberries, ½ cup (C)	37
Blueberries, ½ C	40
Sweet cherries, 10	49
Dried dates, 10	228
Dried figs, 10	477
Grapefruit, pink/red, ½ medium	39
Grapes, 1 C	58
Guava, 1 medium	46
Honeydew, 1 C, cubed	60
Kiwi, 1 medium	46
Mango, 1 medium	135
Nectarine, 1 medium	67
Navel orange, 1 medium	60
Papaya, 1 medium	119
Peach, 1 medium	37
Pear, 1 medium	98
Pineapple, 1 C	76
Plum, 1 medium	36
Dried prunes, 10	201
Seedless raisins, ⅔ C	300
Raspberries, ½ C	30
Strawberries, 1 C	45
Tangerine, 1 medium	37
Watermelon, 1 C, cubed	51

*** If you are counting calories, these charts will help you keep track!	
Vegetable and Serving Size	**Calories**
Alfalfa sprouts, 1 C, raw	10
Artichoke, 1 medium, boiled	150
Asparagus, 6 spears, boiled	22
Beets, ½ C, boiled	37
Broccoli, ½ C, raw	12
Brussels sprouts, ½ C, boiled	30
Green cabbage, ½ C, raw and shredded	9
Carrot, 1 medium, raw	31
Cauliflower, ½ C, raw	13
Celery, 1 stalk, raw	6
Corn, ½ C, boiled	89
Cucumber, ½ C, raw slices	7
Eggplant, ½ C, boiled	11
Green beans, ½ C, boiled	22
Romaine lettuce, ½ C, shredded	4
Mushrooms, ½ C, raw slices	9
Onions, ½ C, raw chopped	30
Parsnips, ½ C, boiled slices	63
Peas, ½ C, frozen, boiled	62
Potato, 1 medium, baked	161
Sweet pepper, ½ C, raw chopped	14
Radishes, 10, raw	8
Spinach, ½ C, raw chopped	6
Summer squash, ½ C, raw slices	13
Tomato, 1, raw	26

If you need to add more sweetness to your juices, feel free to add any of the following:

Honey
Agave Nectar
Blackstrap Molasses
Stevia
Apple Sauce
Vanilla yogurt
Coconut Sugar
Maple Syrup
Maple Sugar
Sugar in the Raw

For a more intense flavor in juice, feel free to add any of the following when juicing:

* Cinnamon
* Citrus (orange, lemon, or lime) juice or zest
* Cloves
* Dried apricots
* Dried cherries
* Fruity red wine
* Ginger, both fresh and ground
* Nutmeg
* Nuts like pistachios, walnuts, hazelnuts, pecans, and almonds
* Star anise
* Toasted coconut flakes
* Vanilla (extract or bean)

Spoiled Rotten

Here, my 'Juicy Friends' are tips on how to store fresh fruits and vegetables so you can enjoy their wonderful flavors, nutritional value and save tons of money.

If your produce rots after just a few days, you might be storing incompatible fruits and veggies together. Those that give off high levels of ethylene gas——a ripening agent——will speed the decay of ethylene-sensitive foods. Keep the two separate.

REFRIGERATE THESE GAS RELEASERS:
- Apples
- Apricots
- Cantaloupe
- Figs
- Honeydew

DON'T REFRIGERATE THESE GAS RELEASERS:
- Avocados
- Bananas, unripe
- Nectarines
- Peaches
- Pears
- Plums
- Tomatoes

KEEP THESE AWAY FROM ALL GAS RELEASERS:
- Bananas, ripe
- Broccoli
- Brussels sprouts
- Cabbage
- Carrots
- Cauliflower
- Cucumbers

- Eggplant
- Lettuce and other leafy greens
- Parsley
- Peas
- Peppers
- Squash
- Sweet potatoes
- Watermelon

EAT FIRST:
- Artichokes
- Asparagus
- Avocados
- Bananas
- Basil
- Broccoli
- Cherries
- Corn
- Green beans
- Mushrooms
- Mustard greens
- Strawberries
- Watercress

EAT NEXT:
- Arugula
- Cucumbers
- Eggplant
- Grapes
- Lettuce
- Lime
- Mesclun
- Pineapple
- Zucchini

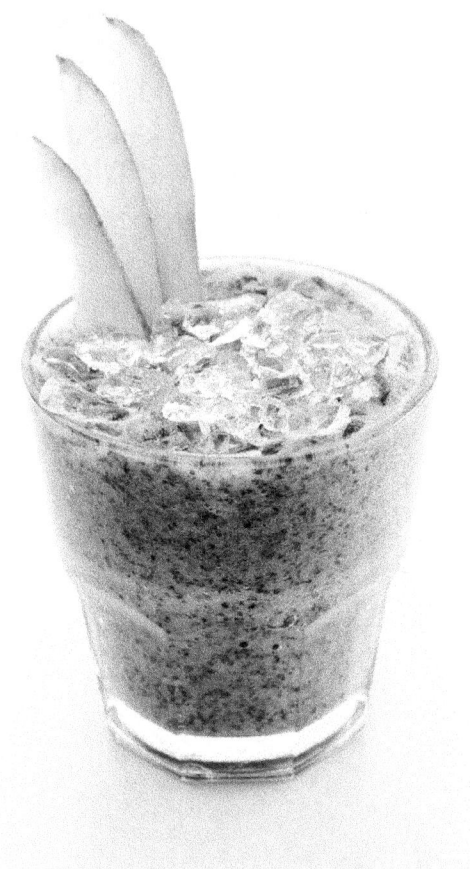

EAT LAST: Weekend
- Apricots
- Bell peppers
- Blueberries
- Brussels sprouts
- Cauliflower
- Grapefruit
- Leeks
- Lemons
- Mint
- Oranges
- Oregano
- Parsley
- Peaches
- Pears
- Plums
- Spinach
- Tomatoes
- Watermelon

AND BEYOND:
- Apples
- Beets
- Cabbage
- Carrots
- Celery
- Garlic
- Onions
- Potatoes
- Winter squash

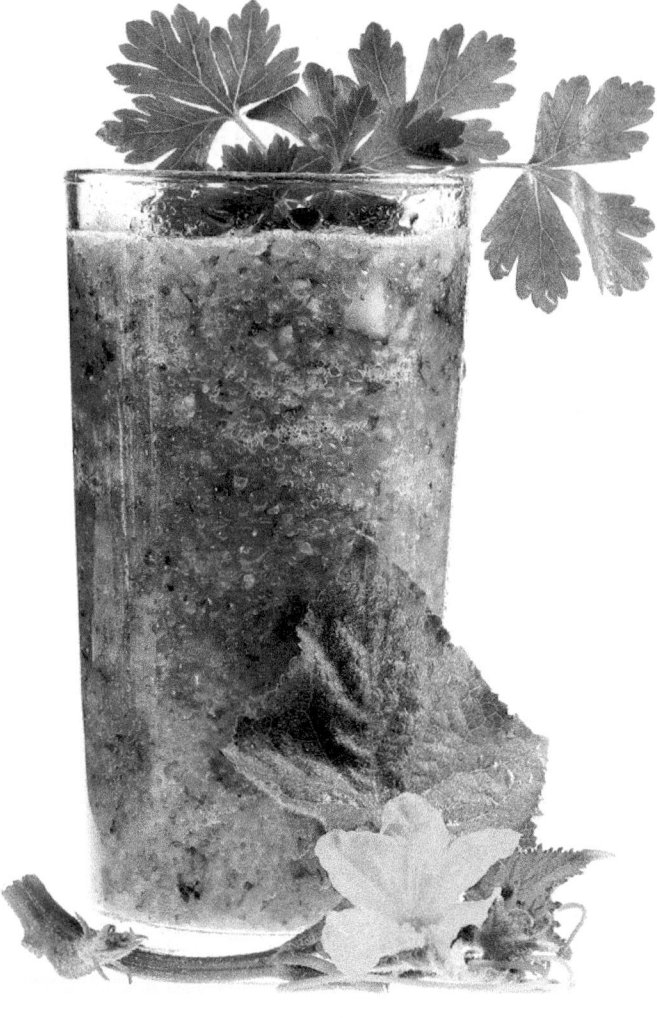

Fresh Vegetable and Fruit Storage Chart			
Fresh Vegetable	Fridge Time	Freezer Time	Storage Tips
Asparagus	2-3 days	8-12 months	Don't wash before refrigerating. Store in crisper.
Brussels sprouts and broccoli	3-5 days	8-12 months	Wrap odorous foods and refrigerate in crisper.
Celery	1-2 weeks	Not recommended	Refrigerate in crisper.
Cauliflower and snap beans	1 week	8-12 months	Wrap odorous foods and refrigerate in crisper.
Carrots, parsnips, beets, radishes and turnips	2 weeks	8-12 months	Remove tops. Wrap odorous foods and refrigerate in crisper.
Eggplant	2 weeks	Not recommended	Store in paper bag in crisper.

Green peas/lima beans	3-5 days	8-12 months	Leave in pods and refrigerate.
Lettuce/other salad greens	1 week	Not recommended	Wash. Drain well. Wrap and refrigerate in crisper.
Mushrooms	3-5 days	Not recommended	Store in paper bag in crisper.
Onions, green	3-5 days	8-12 months	Wrap odorous foods and refrigerate in crisper.
Onions, yellow	2 weeks	Not recommended	In an open paper bag or basket, in a cool dark area, not refrigerated, not directly with potatoes.
Peppers and cucumbers	1 week	8-12 months	Wrap odorous foods and refrigerate in crisper.
Potatoes (new only)	1-2 weeks	Not recommended	Unwashed, in the crisper.

Potatoes (bakers)	1 month	Not recommended	In an open paper bag or basket, in a cool dark area, not refrigerated.
Squash (winter)	1-2 months	Cooked and mashed can be stored 8-12 months	Fresh, store in an open basket in a cool dark, dry area.
Squash (summer)	4-5 days	Slice into rounds, blanch for two minutes, plunge into cold water, drain, and seal in airtight containers. 8-12 months.	Store in plastic bag in crisper drawer four to five days, do not wash until ready to use.
Fresh Fruit			
Apples	1-2 weeks	Only as sauce or sliced for pies	Store apples unwrapped.
Avocadoes	1 week	Not recommended	Ripen on counter before use.
Berries	3-5 days	3-6 months	Do not wash, store in vented

			container/bag.
Cherries	1-2 weeks	Pitted first, 3-6 months	Unwashed, in crisper.
Grapes	1 week	Not recommended	Do not wash, store in vented container/bag.
Melons	1 week	Not recommended	Wrap on counter, store in crisper. Watermelon will not ripen off the vine, store immediately.
Peaches/nectarines	1 week	3-6 months	Store in vented container/bag.

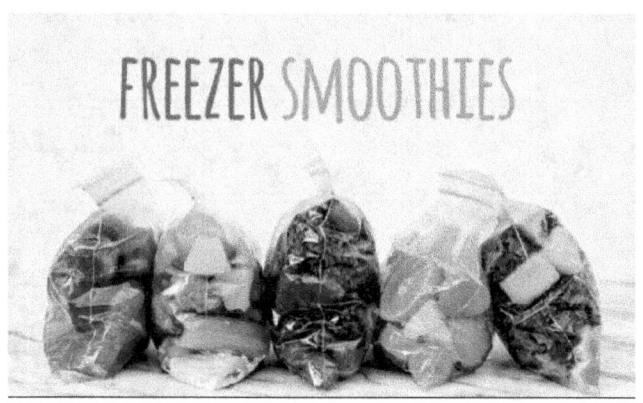

FREEZER SMOOTHIES

Smoothies make a satisfying way to refuel after working out, a great quick breakfast when you're on the go, a refreshing afternoon pick me up and/or a meal replacement. Freezing fresh fruit for smoothies not only retains most of their nutritional properties but by creating individual serving smoothie bags, it's a convenient time saver!

You're not exactly reaching in your freezer and pulling out a ready-made smoothie. Although, boy, wouldn't that be nice! It's more along the lines of having all the fruit your smoothie recipe calls for, prepared and stored in one convenient bag. No more fumbling through the freezer for three different bags of fruit, then trying to find the spinach that's buried somewhere in the back of the fridge.

Prepping your smoothies shaves off precious extra minutes in your daily routine. You can even prep the smoothies before hand for loved ones that may need extra nourishment but find cutting fruits and vegetables to be a challenge. Just cut, bag it and freeze it! A highly nutritious smoothie is waiting for you to indulge in, right inside your freezer for whenever your body needs it.

JUiCYLIFE
with Jenny Patrizia

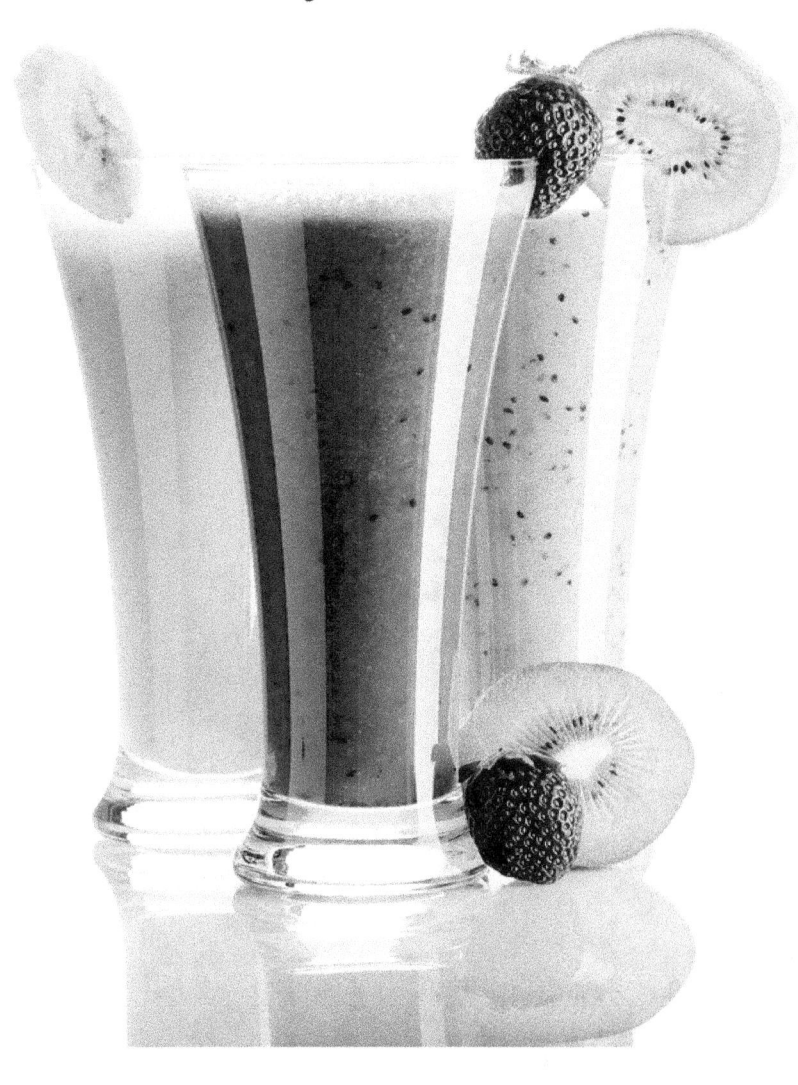

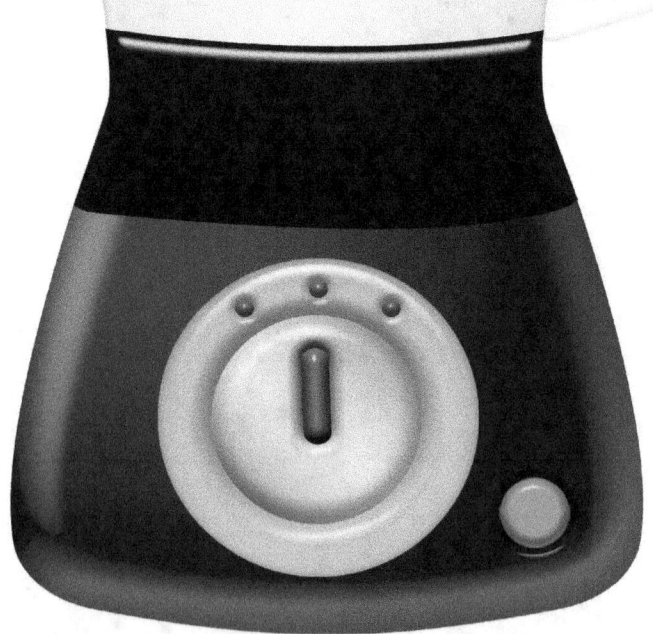

Juice for Acid Reflux

½ Cup of Ice
2 Cups of 1% Milk
2 Bananas
1 Cup of Vanilla Yogurt
½ tbsp Ginger
2 tbsp of Honey
1 tbsp of Dry Oats

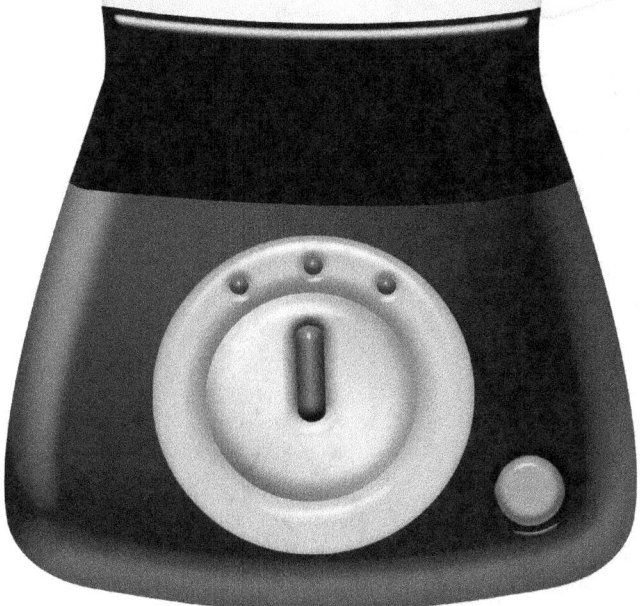

Juice for Acne

2 Cups of Water
½ Cup of Spinach
½ Cup of Lettuce
2 Stalks of Celery
1 Pear, Cubed
1tbsp of Lemon
1 Banana
1 Green Apple
½ Cucumber
2 Kale Leaves
1 tsp of Flaxseed
1 Walnut, Unshelled

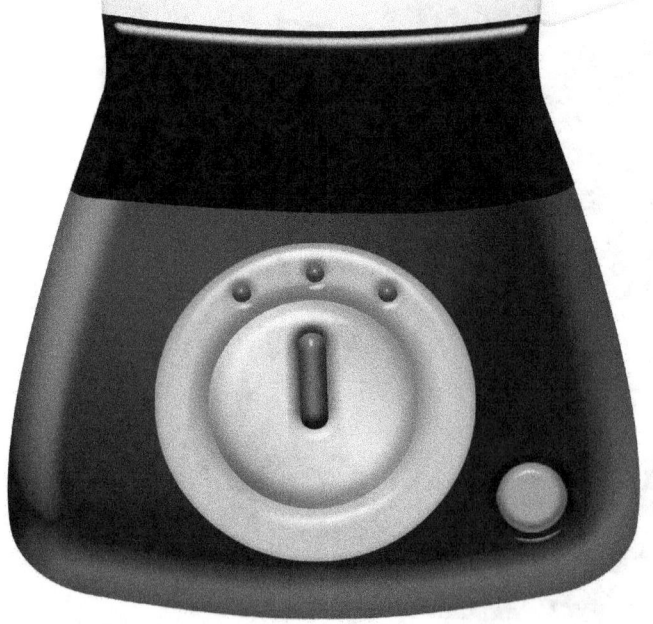

Juice for ADHD

- ½ Cup Melon, Cubed
- ½ Cup of Strawberries
- 1/3 Cup of Low-Fat Milk
- ¼ Cup of Evaporated Milk
- 2 tbsp Flaxseed, Powder
- 1 Cup of Ice
- 1 tbsp of Agave
- 5 Almonds, Unsalted
- 7 Blueberries

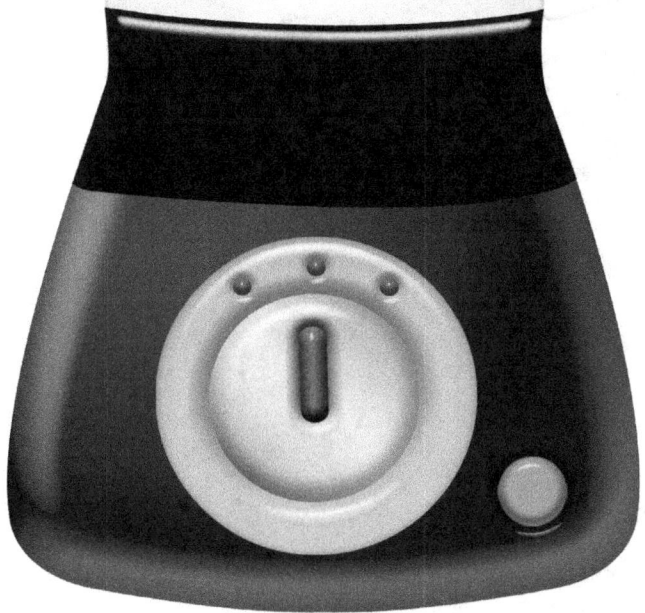

Juice for Allergies

1 Cup of Beets, Sliced
2 Celery Stalks
½ Cup of Cabbage
2 Carrots
1 Cup of Orange Juice
1 Cup of Lettuce
1 Cup of Spinach
1 tsp Cinnamon
1 tsp of Honey
1 Kiwi, Peeled and Sliced

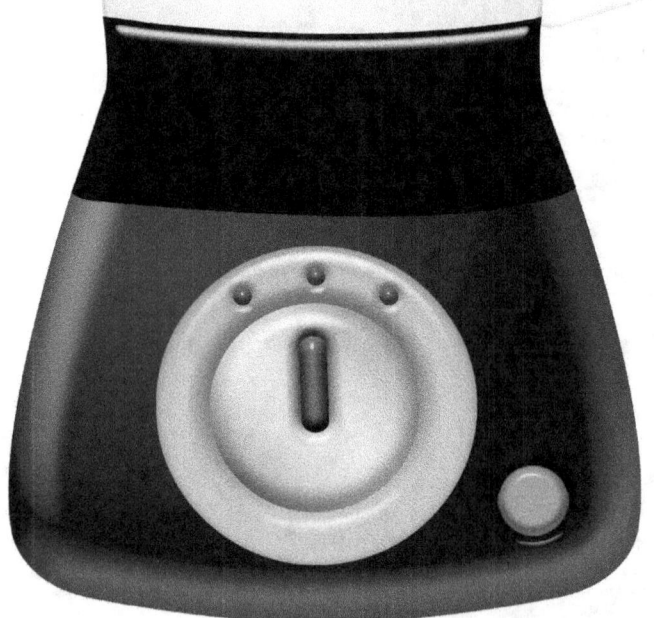

Juice for Anemia

1 Cup of Spinach
1 Cup of Berries
1 Banana
1 tbsp Parsley
1 Cup of Almond Milk
1 Cup Vanilla Yogurt
6 Raisins
½ tbsp. Pumpkin Seeds
½ tsp Wheat Germ
½ Cup of Apricots, Pitted

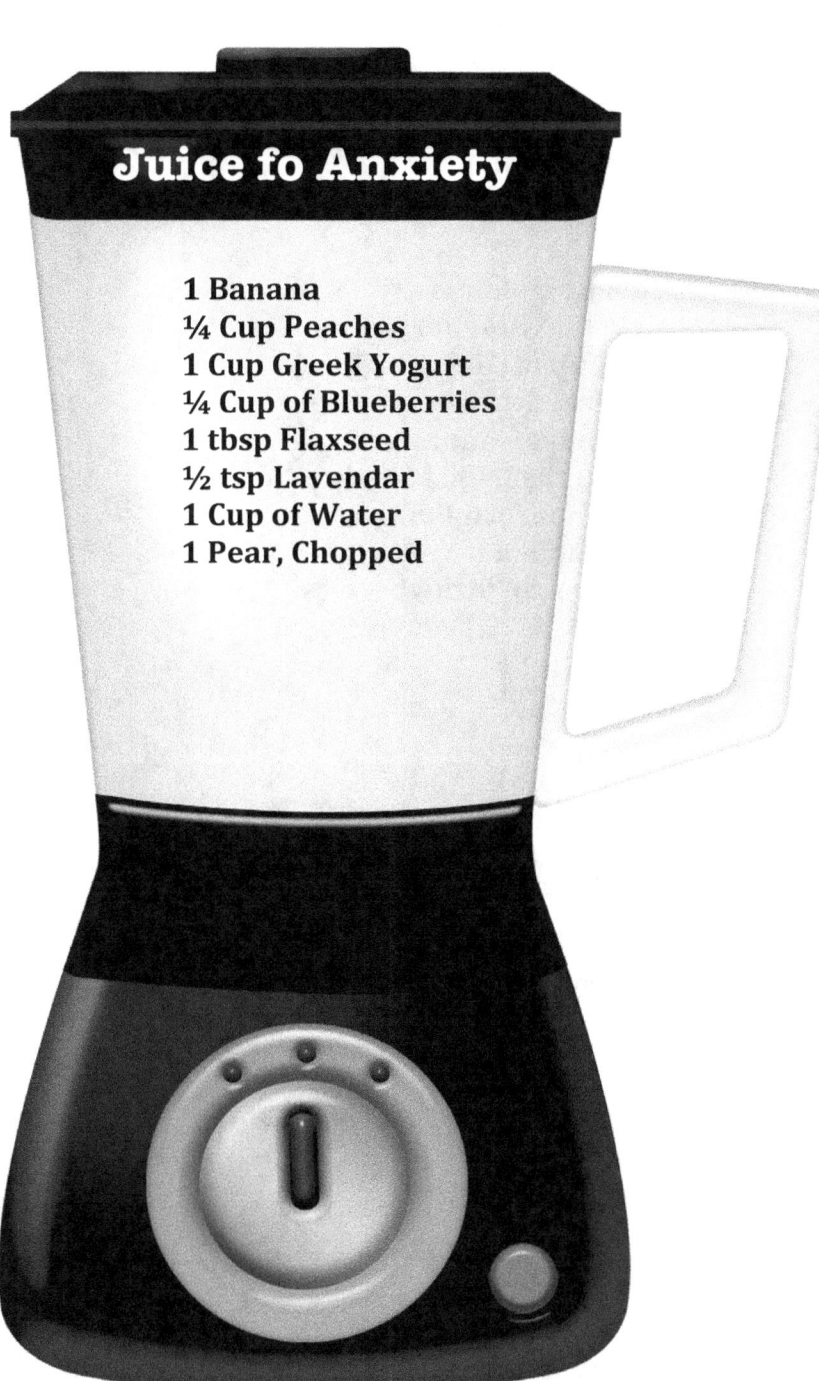

Juice fo Anxiety

1 Banana
¼ Cup Peaches
1 Cup Greek Yogurt
¼ Cup of Blueberries
1 tbsp Flaxseed
½ tsp Lavendar
1 Cup of Water
1 Pear, Chopped

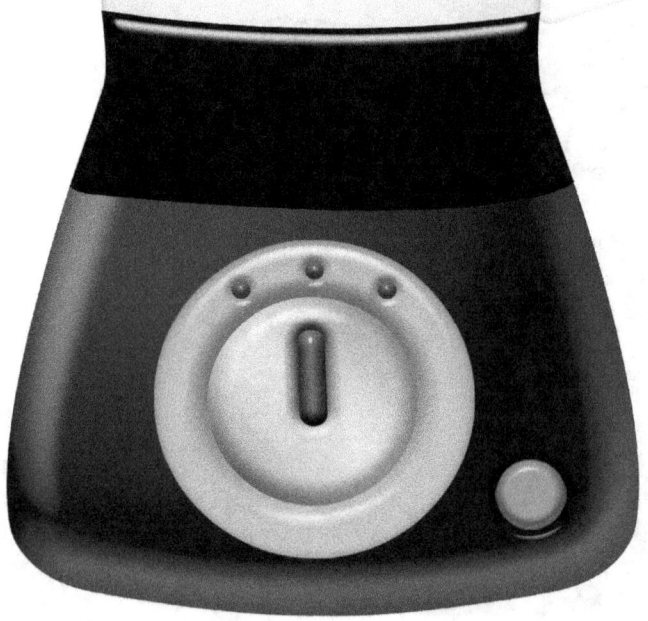

Juice for the Arteries

- ½ Cup of Oats
- ½ Cup Blueberries
- 1 Cup of Almond Milk
- 1 Cup Strawberry Yogurt
- 1 Cup of Spinach
- 1 ½ tbsp. Chia Seeds
- 3 ½ oz Acai Berries
- 1 Banana
- 5 Frozen Strawberries

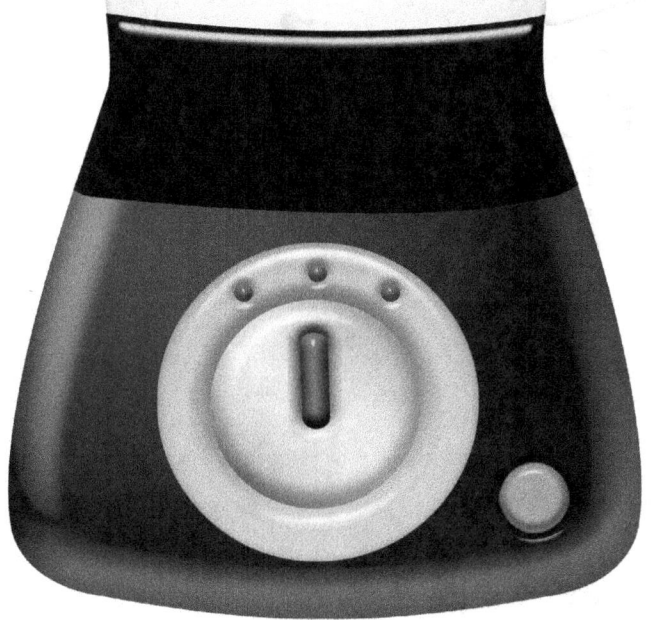

Juice for Arthritis

½ Cup Green Tea
1 ½ Cups Pineapple, Cubed
2 Large Carrots, Chopped
2 tbsp Chia Seeds
½ tsp of Fresh Ginger
2 Cups Spinach
1 Cup of Orange Juice

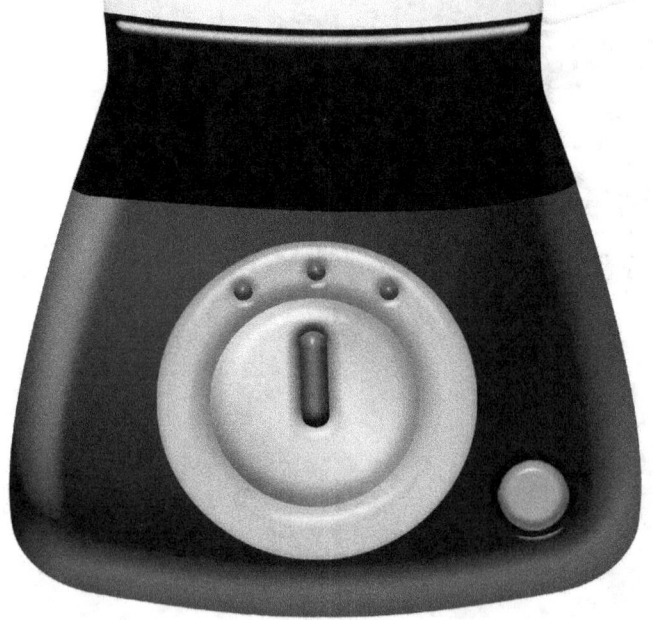

Juice for Asthma

3 Cups of Watermelon
1 Cup of Non-Fat Yogurt
½ Cup of Green Tea
1 tbsp of Mint, Chopped
1 tbsp Lemon Juice
½ Cup of Coconut Water
1 tbsp of Flaxseed Powder

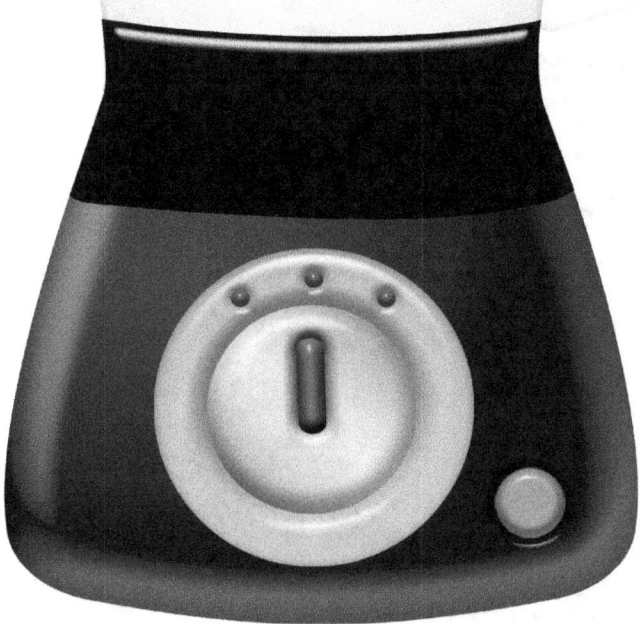

Juice for Autism

¾ Cups Organic Berries
¾ Cups Organic Frozen Peaches
¼ Cup Organic Broccoli Florets
1 Cup Organic Peach Yogurt
¼ Cup Organic Orange Juice
1 tbsp Lemon Juice
1 Cup Natural Mango Juice

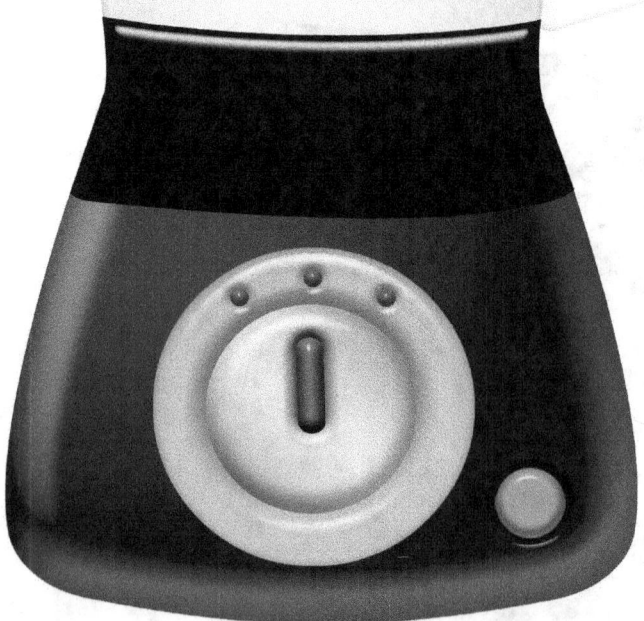

Juice for Bad Breath

1 Cup of Kale
1 Cup Spinach
1 Peach, Sliced & Pitted
1 tbsp Parsley
1 tbsp Mint, chopped
1 tsp of Ginger
1 Cup of Pineapple Juice
1 Cup of Orange Juice

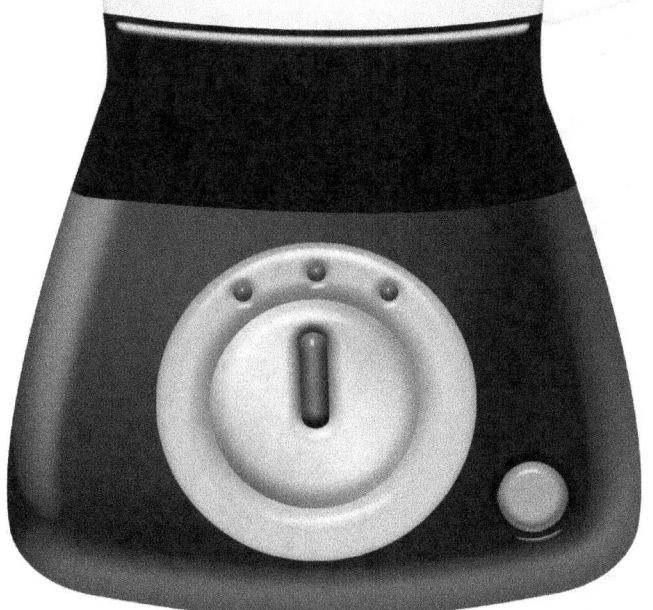

Juice for Blood Pressure

½ Cup of Kiwi, Sliced
1 Cup of Melon
1 Cup Blueberries
½ Cup Spinach
1 Banana
1 Cup Almond Milk
1 Cup Non-Fat Yogurt
½ Avocado, Sliced
Dash of Cinnamon
2 Basil Leaves

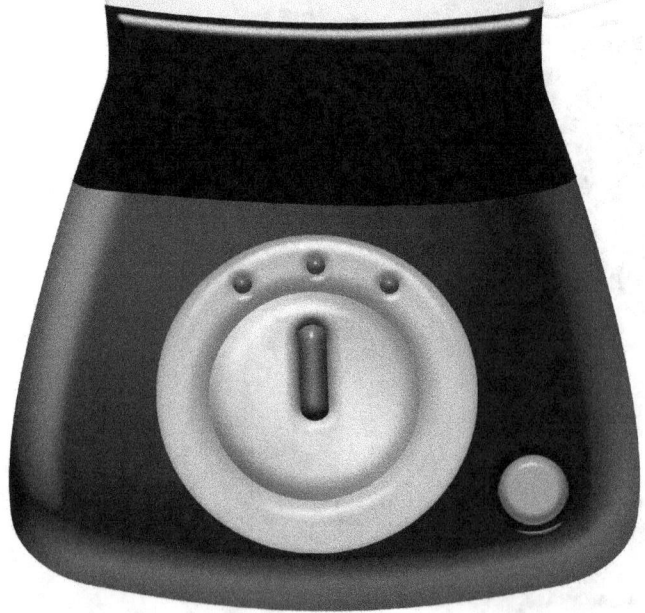

Juice for Body Pains

1 Cup of Watercress
2 Bananas, Frozen
1 Cup of Coconut Water
1 Cup of Pineapple Juice
½ tbsp of Coffee Grounds
1 Pear, Cubed
Dash of Tumeric
Dash of Ginger

People with gallbladder disease should avoid using turmeric

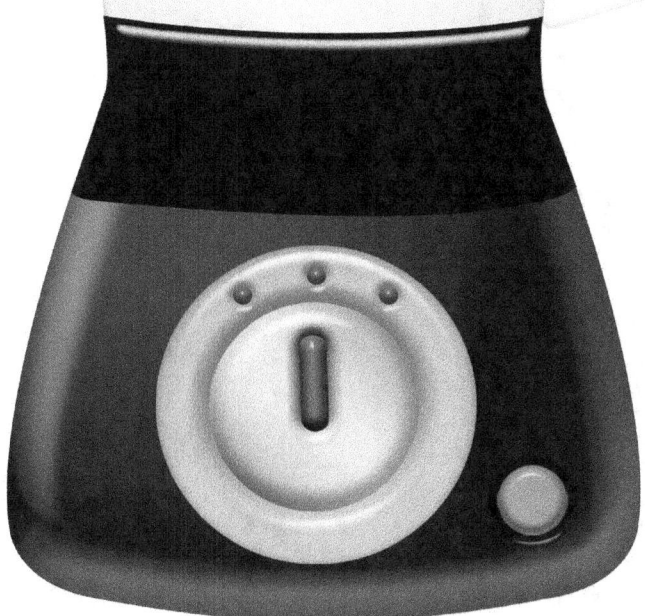

Juice for Fuller Breasts

2 Cups of Papaya, Cubed
½ Cup of Almond Milk
5 Pitted Cherries
1 Pinch of Licorice
1 Cup of Soy Milk
Dash of Fennel Seeds
1 Apple, Sliced
3 tbsp of Rice

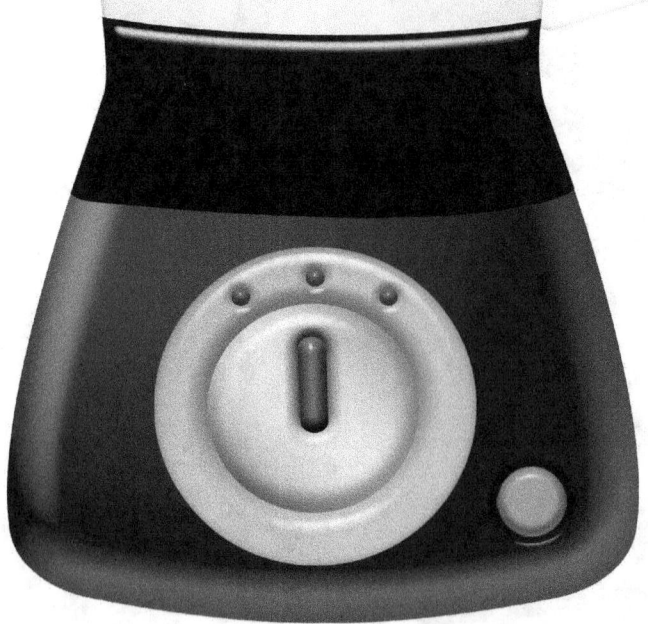

Juice for Breastfeeding

1 Cup of Spinach
2 tbsp of Oats
2 tbsp Flaxseed Seeds
1 Banana
1/3 Cup Peach, Pitted
1 tbsp Peanut Butter
1/3 Cup of Mangos
½ Cup Greek Yogurt
1/3 Cup Soy Milk
½ tbsp Cacao Powder

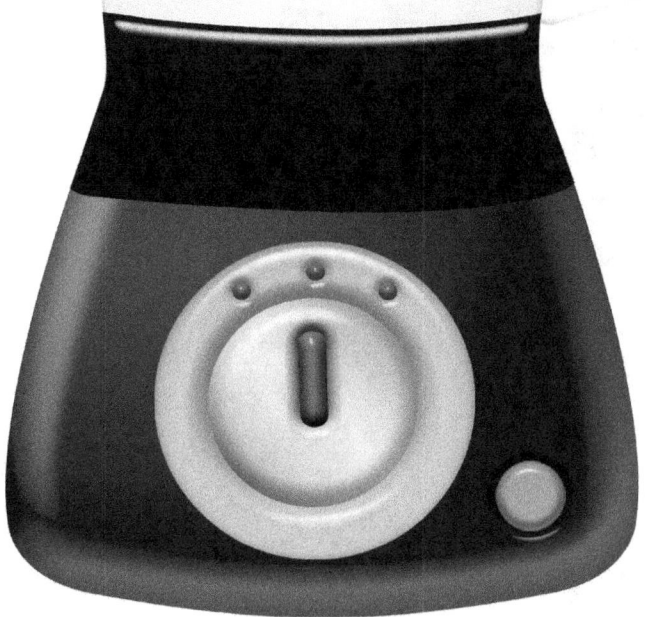

Juice for Bronchitis

1 Cup of Berries
3 Celery Stalks
½ Cup of Goji Berries
1 tbsp of Lemon Juice
Pinch of Apple Vinegar
½ tbsp of Ginger
1 tsp of Cinnamon
Pinch of Cayenne Powder
1/3 cup Cranberry Juice
½ cup Grape Juice

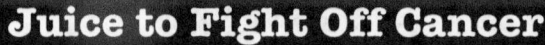

Juice to Fight Off Cancer

1 Cup of Alkaline Water
2 tbsp Chia Seeds
1 Cup of Raspberries
1 Organic Banana
1 Cup Organic Broccoli
1 cup of Oats, Raw
2 tbsp of Sunflower Seeds
½ Cup of Raisins or Grapes
1 Cup Green Tea
1 Apple, Sliced

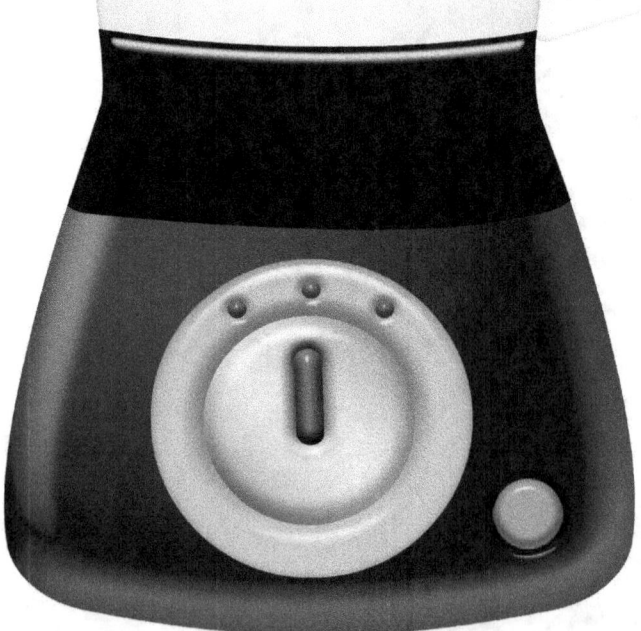

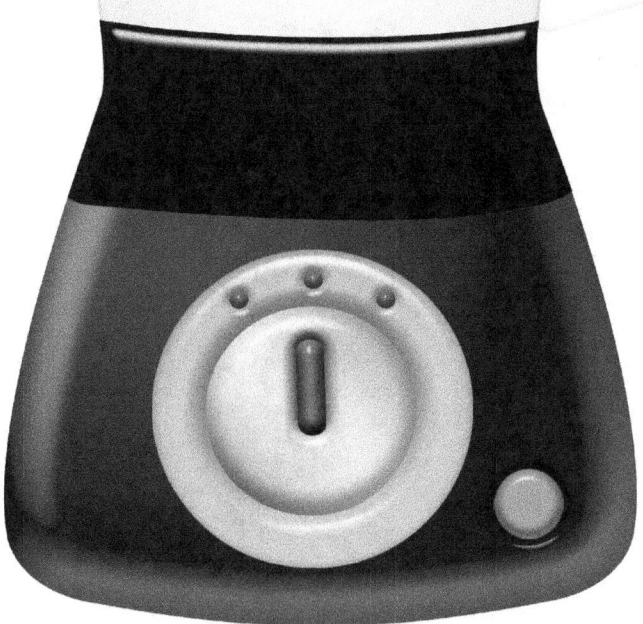

Juice to Reduce Cellulite

2 Cups of Water
1 Cup of Blueberries
5 Strawberries
1 tbsp Ginger
1 Banana
1 Cup of Pineapple
1 Cup of Papaya
½ tsp Cinnamon
1 Cup Spinach

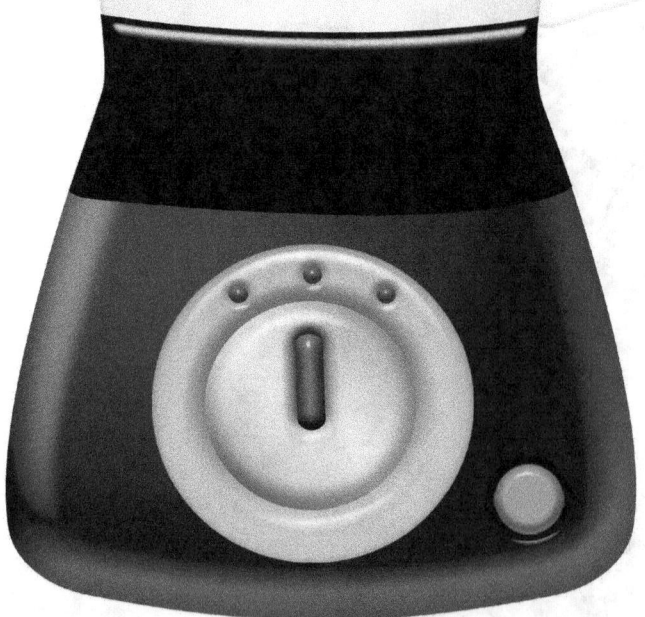

Juice for Cholesterol

1 Cup of Yogurt, Plain
5 Ice Cubes
6 Strawberries
2 Kiwis, No Skin
1 Cup of Pineapple, Cubed
1 Banana
½ Green Pear
1 tbsp Flaxseed Powder
2 tbsp Oats
1tsp Soybean Oil
Dash of Tumeric

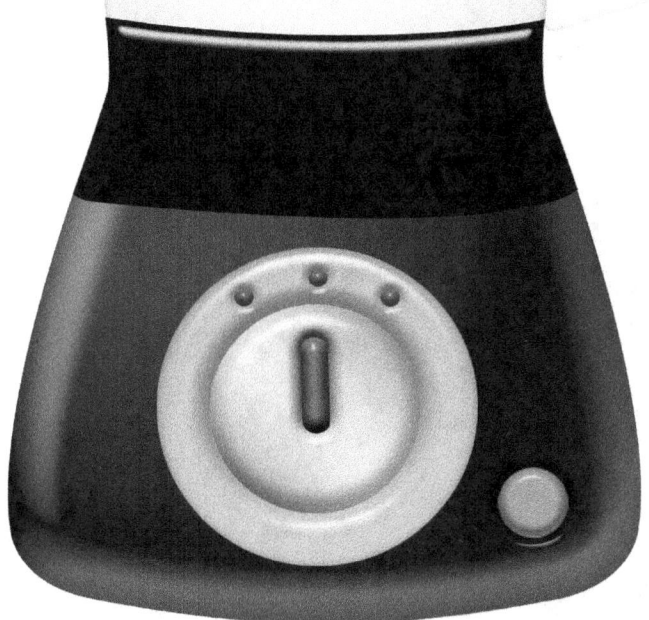

Juice for the Circulation

½ Cup of Cranberry Juice
1 Banana
6 Strawberries
½ Greek Yogurt, Blueberry
1 Orange, Peeled
2 (6 oz) Dark Chocolate
1/3 Cup Green Tea

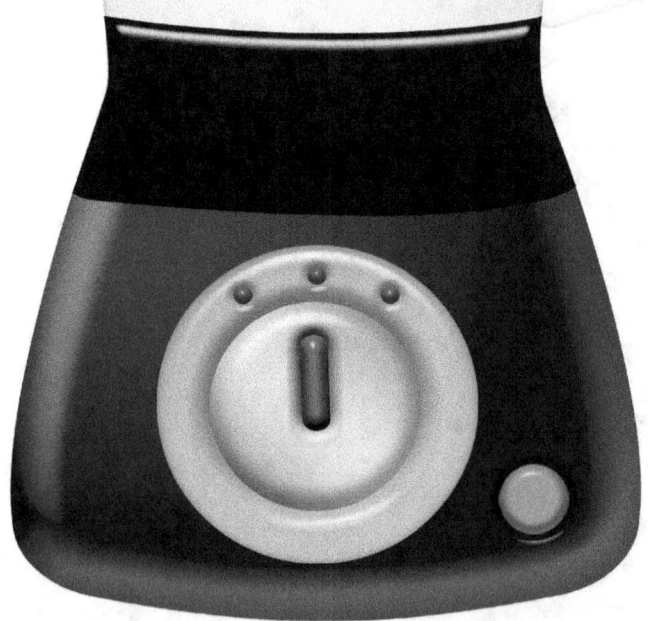

Juice to Fight off a Cold

1 Cup of Strawberries
1 Orange, Peeled
3 Kale Leaves
½ Cup of Pineapple Juice
1 tbsp of Honey
½ Cup of Ice
1 tsp of Lemon Juice
1 Vitamin C 500 mg Tablet

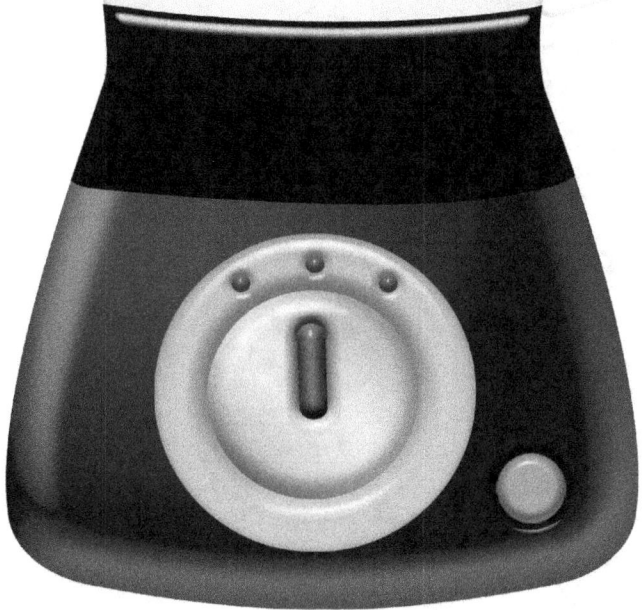

Juice for Congestion

3 Stalks of Celery
1/4 Cup of Onions, Chopped
1 Garlic Clove
1 Broccoli Bundle
1 Red Apple
2 Cup of White Grape Juice
1 Cup Seedless Red Grapes
1 tbsp of Honey
1 tsp of Cinnamon

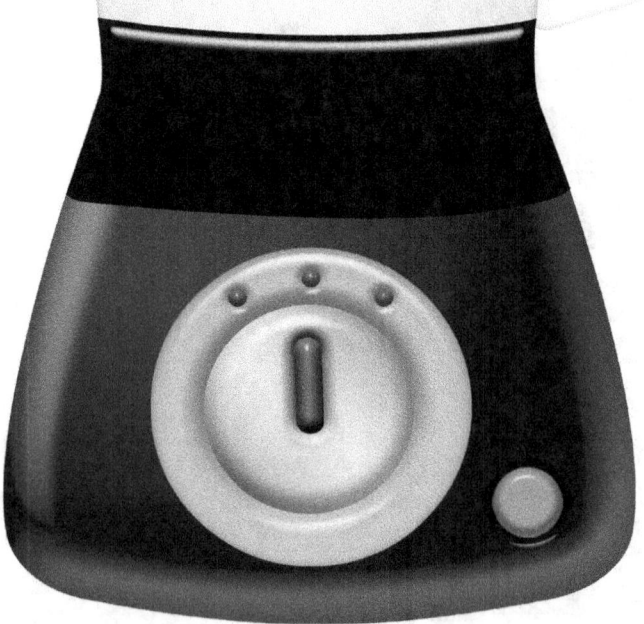

Juice for Constipation

½ Cup of Prune Juice
1 Cup of Ice Cubes
½ Cup of Coconut Milk
¼ Cup Mixed Frozen Berries
2 Slices of Papaya
½ Cup of Oats
1 Vanilla Probiotic Yogurt

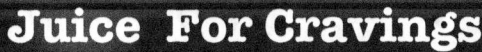

Juice For Cravings

1/3 Cup of Mango, Cubed
1 Cup Frozen Strawberries
½ Cup Spinach
2 Cups Coconut Water
1 tbsp Agave
1 tbsp Chia Seed
1 tbsp Hemp Protein Powder
1 tbsp Cacao

Hemp Protein resembles the protein found in human blood and therefore it is the easiest type of protein to digest. Hemp contains less than 0.3% THC whereas US law defines hemp as all parts of any Cannabis Sativa plant containing NO psychoactive properties. Hemp protein contains 21 known amino acids, 9 of which our bodies cannot produce on our own. It also contains Omega Fatty Acids and Fiber.

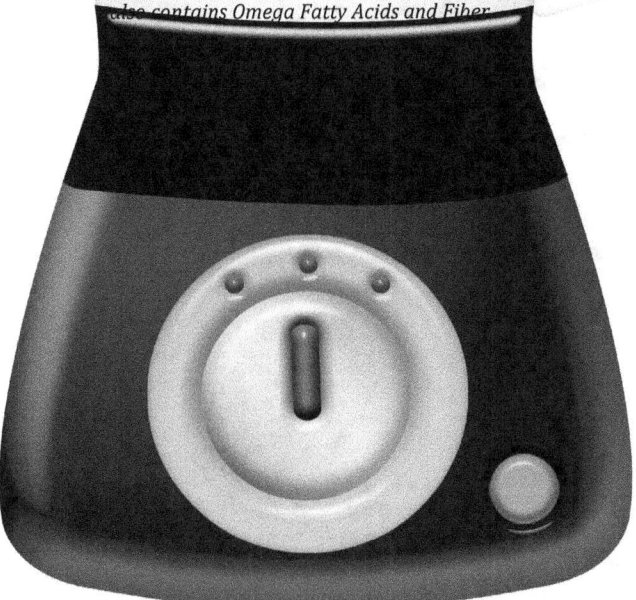

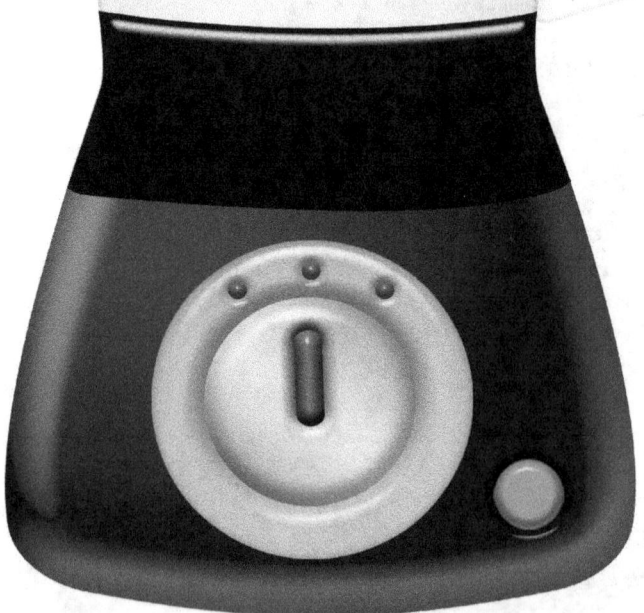

Juice for Dehydration

3 Apricots, Pitted
7 Strawberries
1 Cup Carrot Juice
1 Cup of Orange Juice
1 tbsp of Flaxseed Powder
1 Beet, Sliced
1 slice of Watermelon
¼ Cup Electrolyte Juice

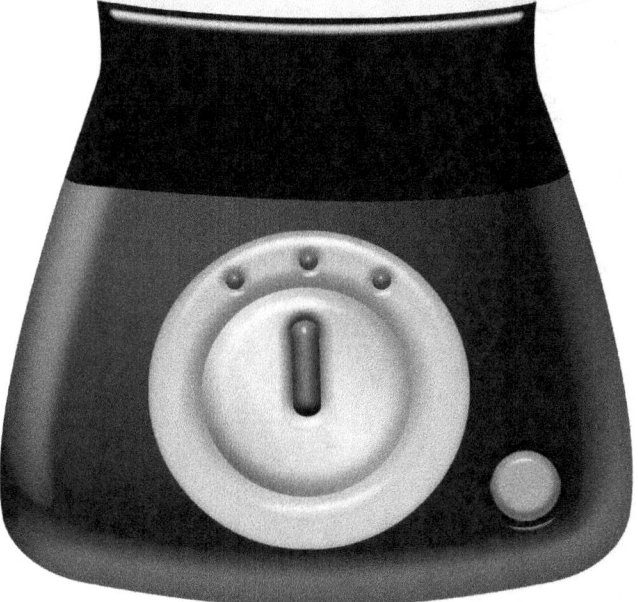

Juice for Ebola

½ Cup Dried Apricots
½ Cup Dried Dates
2 tbsp Chickpeas
Handulll of Alfalfa Sprouts
1 Cup of Coconut Milk
1 Garcinia Kola Capsule
1 Vitamin C 500 mg Tablet
½ tbsp. Fiber Powder
1 tbsp Whey Protein Powder

Chief Medical Officer of John F Kennedy Memorial Hospital, Dr. Billy Johnson, says Ebola can be defeated in the body when it meets the bodies build up with more protein, estradiol and Fiber in our systems.

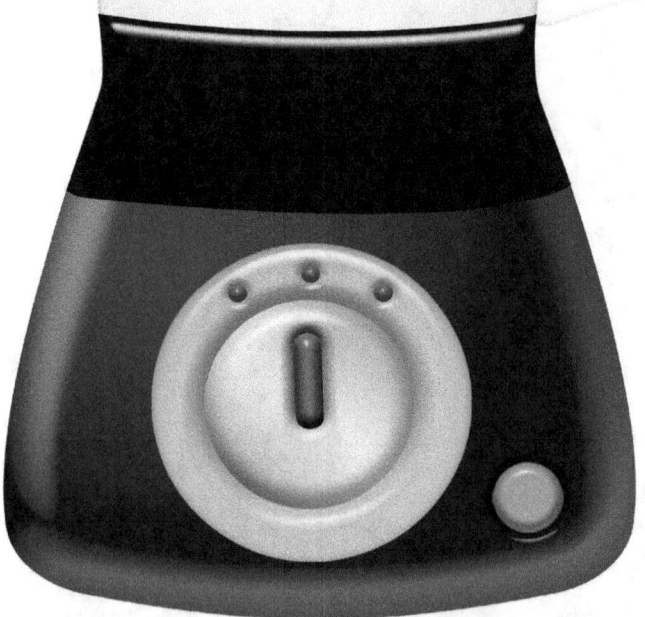

Juice for Depression

- ½ Cup of Pineapple
- 1 Cup Flax Milk
- 1 Organic Banana
- 1 Red Apple, Sliced
- 1 Orange, Peeled
- 1 Cup of Spinach
- ½ Cup of Kale
- 1 tsp of Ground Chia Seeds
- 1 tsp of Spirulina Powder
- 1 tsp of Rice Protein Powder

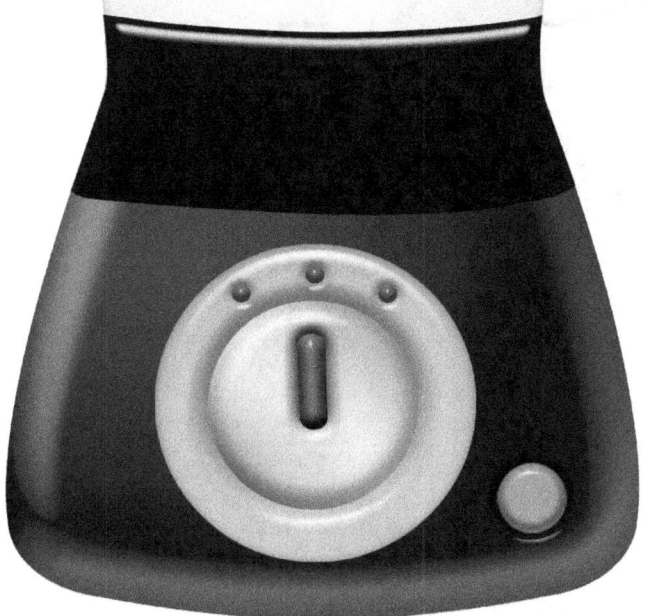

Juice to Detox the Body

½ tbsp of Honey
¼ Cup of Mixed Herbs
(Mint, Basil, Tarragon)
1 ½ cups Berry Mix
1/2 Cup Coconut Milk
1 cup Purified Water
1/8 cup rolled oats
½ Apple
Dash of Chia Seeds

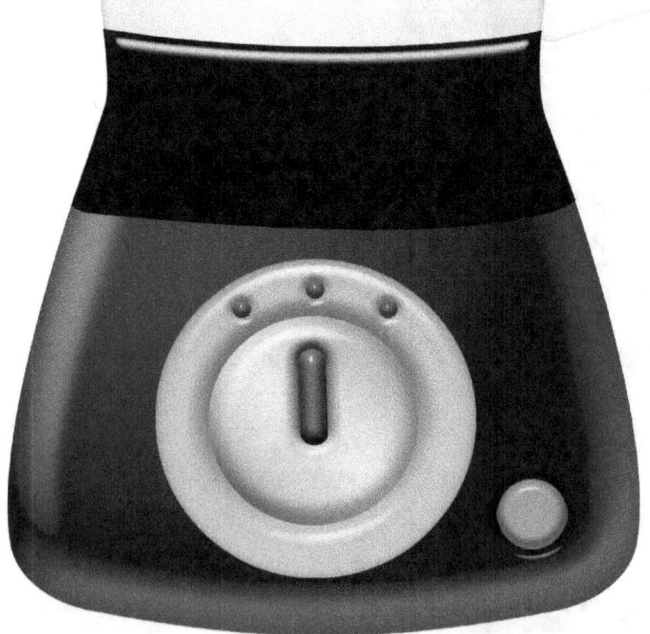

Juice for Diabetes

1/2 Almond Milk
1 tsp Cinnamon
1/2 Cup of Nonfat Greek Yogurt
1/2 Banana, Peeled
1/2 Cup Unsweetened Blueberries
1/2 Cup of Oatmeal, Precooked
1/4 Cup of Almonds, Unsalted
¼ Cup Of Walnuts, Unsalted

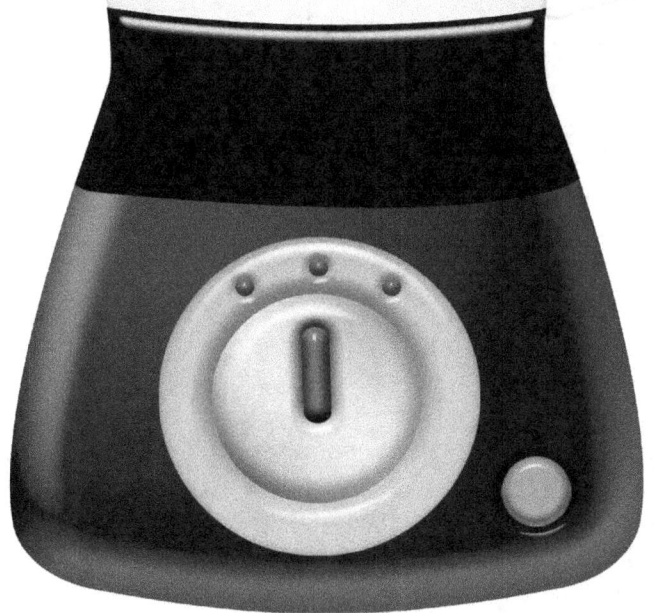

Juice for Dizziness

1 Lemon
½ Apple
½ Banana
3 tbsp Orange Juice
5 Strawberries
1 cup of Pineapple Chunks
½ Cup of Vanilla Yogurt
2 cups of Soy Milk
1 B-Complex Vitamin
1 (500mg) Vitamin C Chewable
1 tsp of Ginger

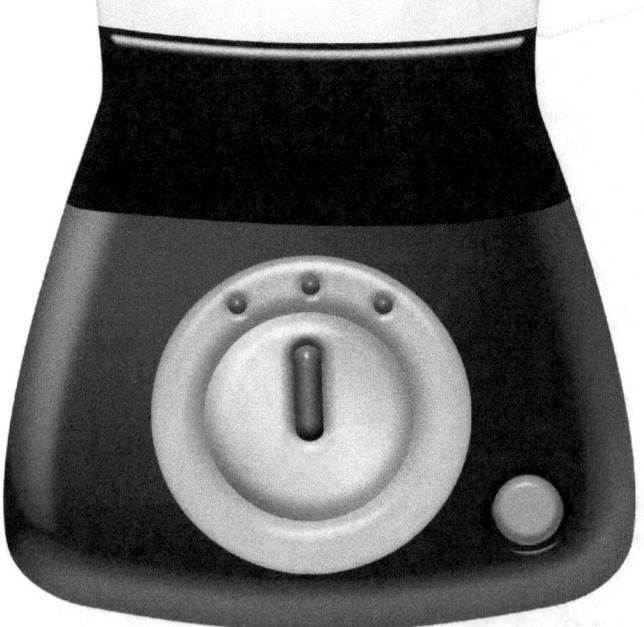

Juice for Ear Infections

1 Tomato
2 tbsp of Onions
1 Garlic Clove
2 Cup of Chicken Soup
4 Broccoli Stubs
½ Cups of Spinach

Juice for Eczema

Half of a Large Avocado
2 Kiwifruit, Peeled
1 tbsp of Coconut Oil
½ Cucumber
2 Branches of Parsley
1 Carrot
1 tbsp Flaxseed
1 Beet
1 tsp Ginger
1 tsp Amla Powder
½ Cup of Hemp Milk

Helps decrease inflammation
Helps promote skin repair

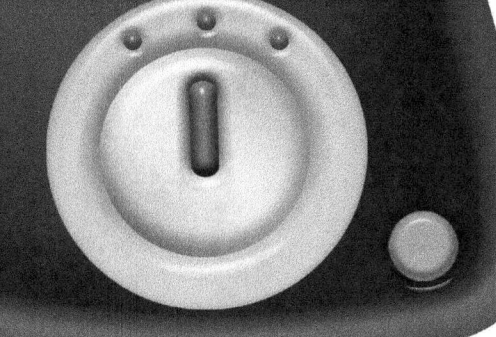

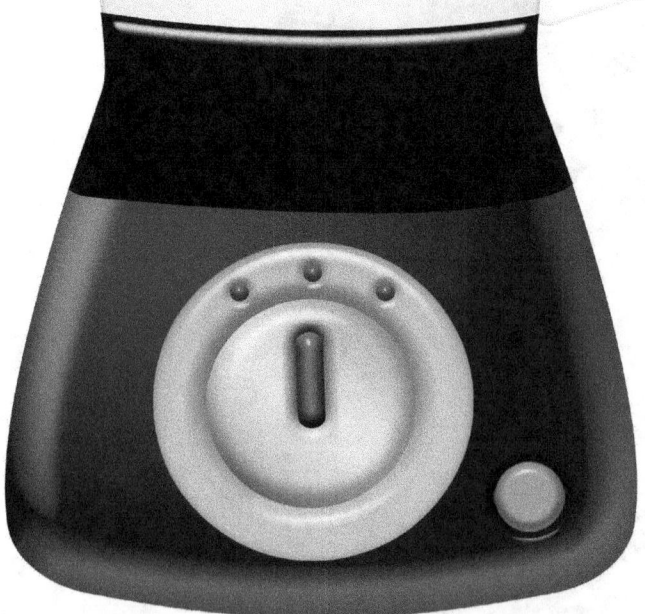

Juice for Energy

1 Cup of Rice, Cooked
1 Cup of Soy Milk
1 Cup Raspberrries
¼ Can Pumpkin
½ Cup of Vanilla Yogurt
½ Frozen Banana
4 ice cubes
1 tbsp Protein Powder
½ tbsp of Cacao Powder

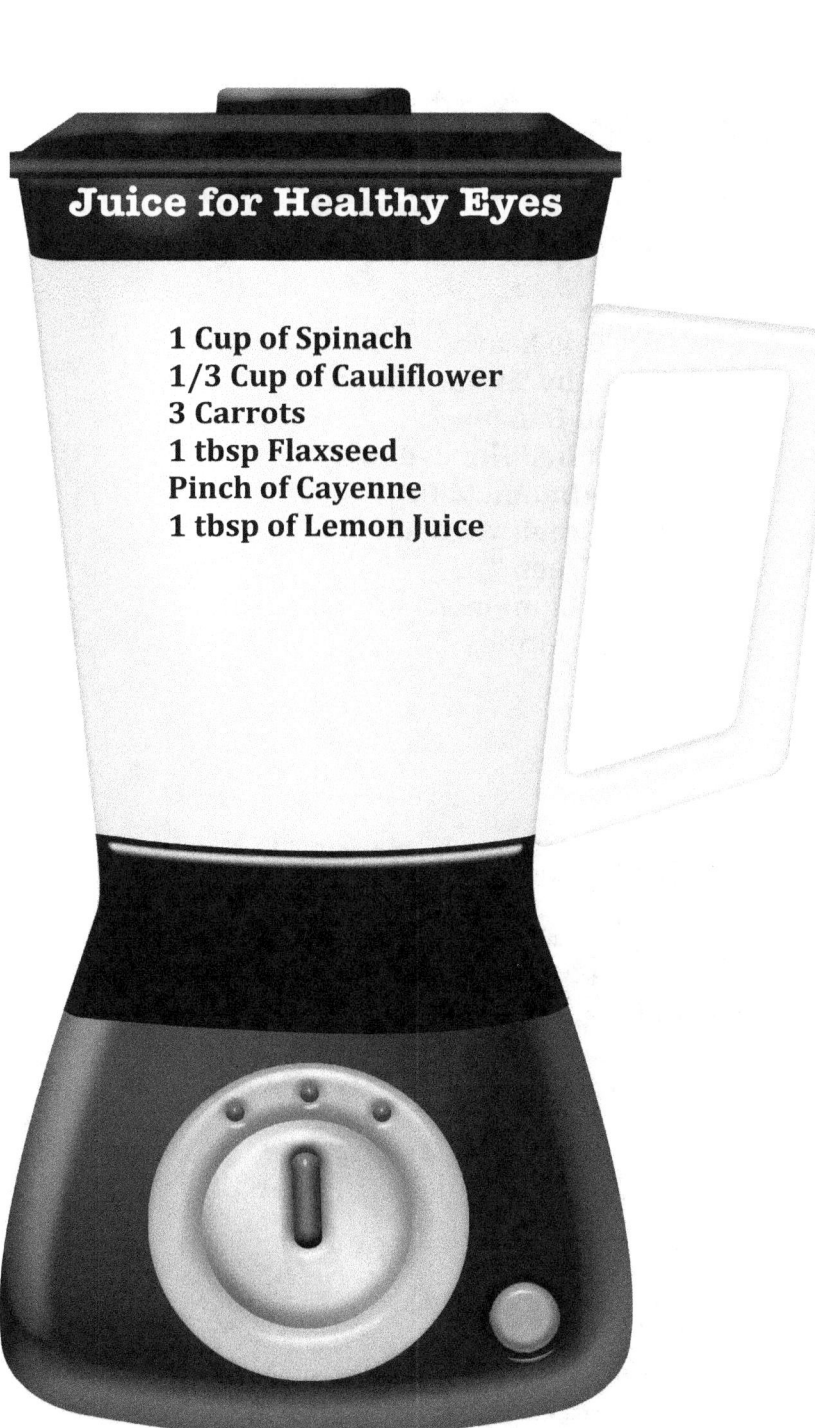

Juice for Healthy Eyes

1 Cup of Spinach
1/3 Cup of Cauliflower
3 Carrots
1 tbsp Flaxseed
Pinch of Cayenne
1 tbsp of Lemon Juice

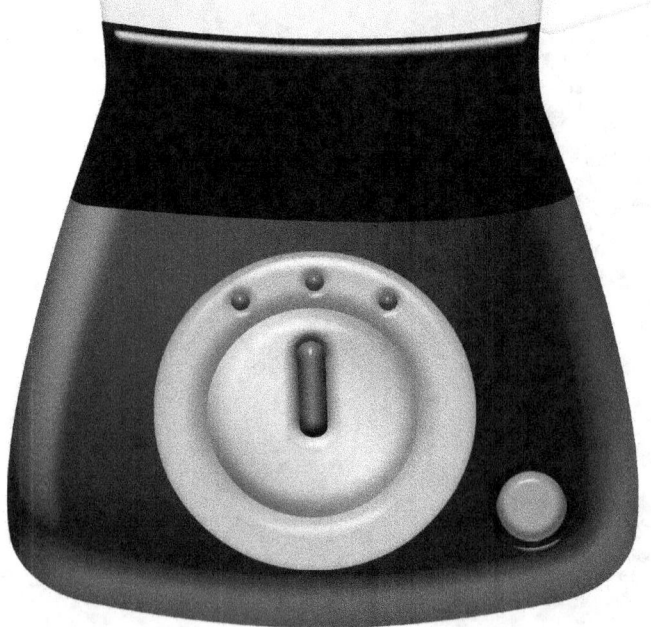

Juice to Burn Fat

1 Cup Kale Leaves
1 Cup Baby Spinach Leaves
1 Frozen Banana
1 Cup Cubed Honeydew Melon
½ Cup Almond Milk
½ Cup Greek Yogurt
½ Cup Green Tea
Dash of Cinnamon
Dash of Nutmeg

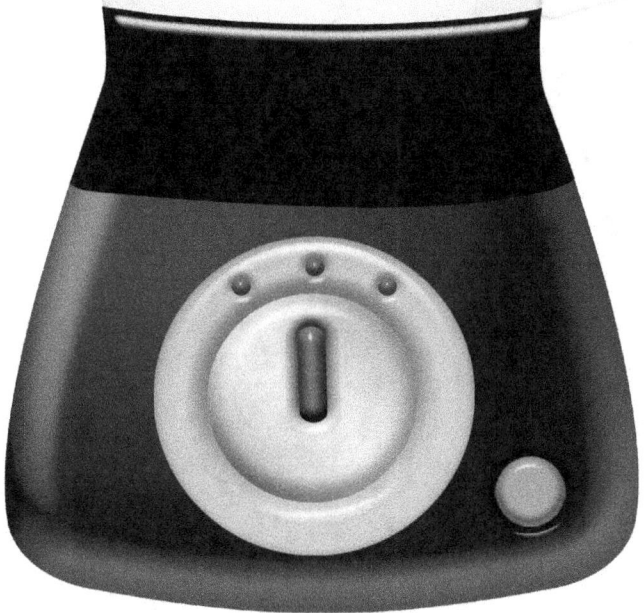

Juice for Fertility

1 tbsp Royal Jelly
½ Cup Mangoes
½ Cup Peach, Sliced
1 Banana
½ Cup Almond Milk
1 Peach Yogurt
2 Shots of Wheatgrass
Dash of Maca Root Powder

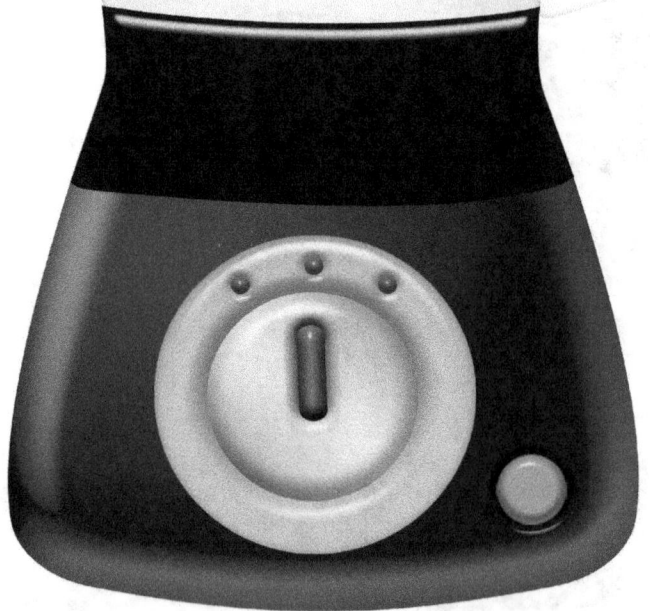

Juice for Fever

1 tbsp Lemon Juice
2 Oranges, Peeled
½ Grapefruit
3 Slices of Pineapple
2 Kiwis, Peeled
Slice of Watermelon
1 tsp Rosemary
Dash of Licorice Powder

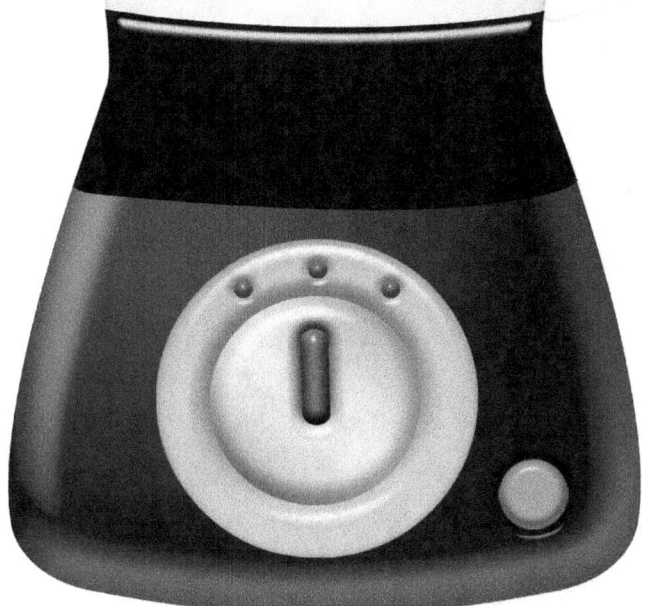

Juice to Relieve Gas

Pinch of Bicarbonate Soda
1 Cup Chamomile Tea
Yogurt with live/active cultures
1 tbsp Wheat Powder
¼ Cup Alfalfa
½ Cup of Water
2 tsp Vanilla Extract
1 tbsp Agave

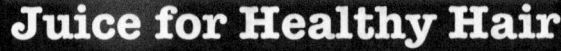

Juice for Healthy Hair

1 tbsp Maple Syrup
2 tbsp Quinoa Grains
1 tsp of Wheat Germ
1 tsp Yeast
1 Egg, Raw
½ Avocado
4 oz Mango Juice
4 oz Soy Milk

Contains Iron, Vitamin C, Protein,
Niacin, Zinc & Biotin for hair growth.

Warning: This juice contains
raw eggs and should consult
a doctor before drinking.

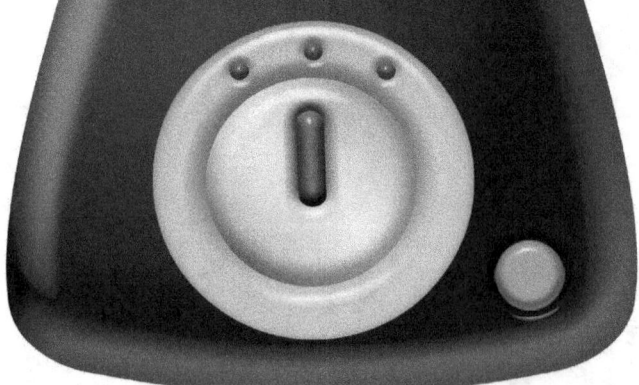

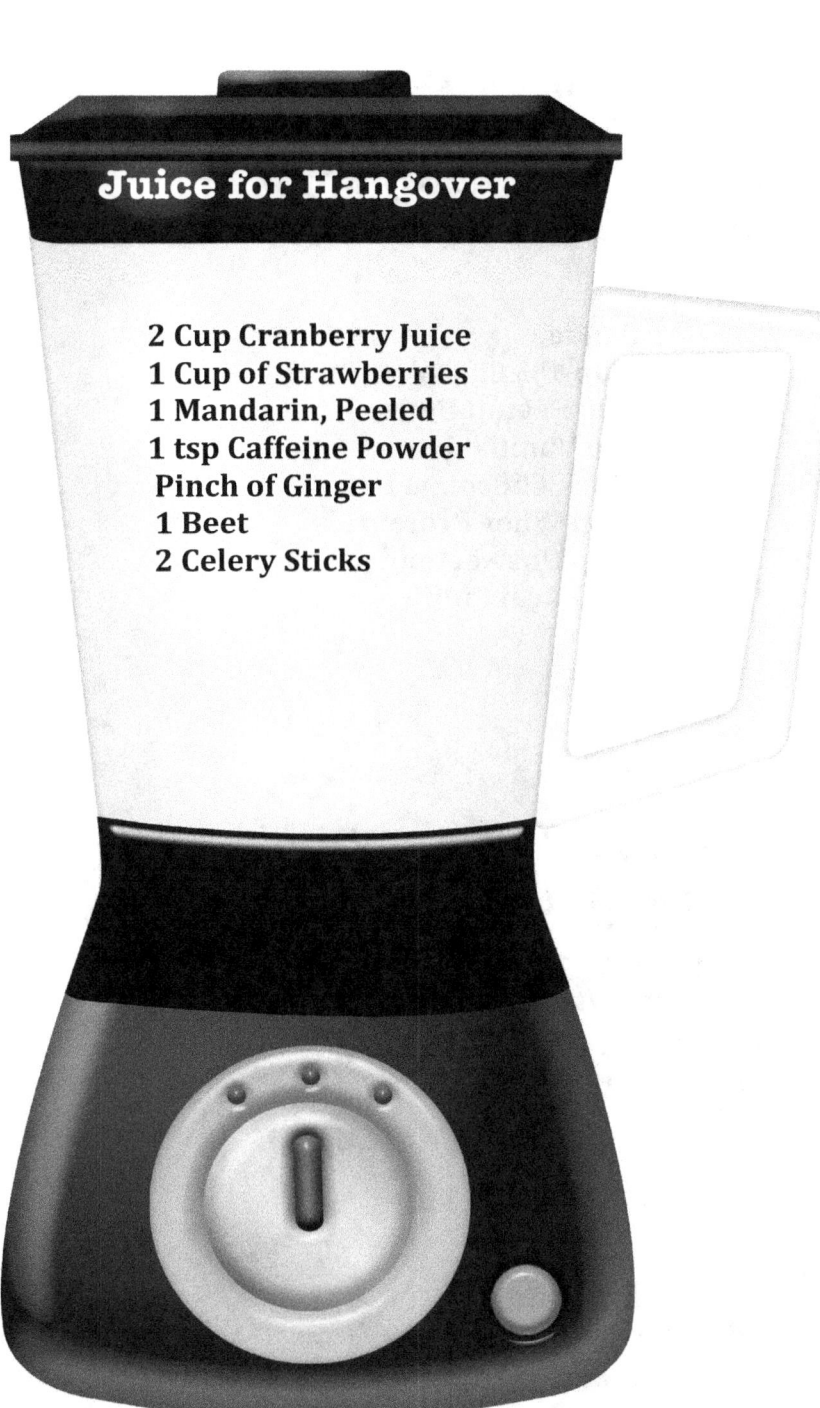

Juice for Hangover

2 Cup Cranberry Juice
1 Cup of Strawberries
1 Mandarin, Peeled
1 tsp Caffeine Powder
Pinch of Ginger
1 Beet
2 Celery Sticks

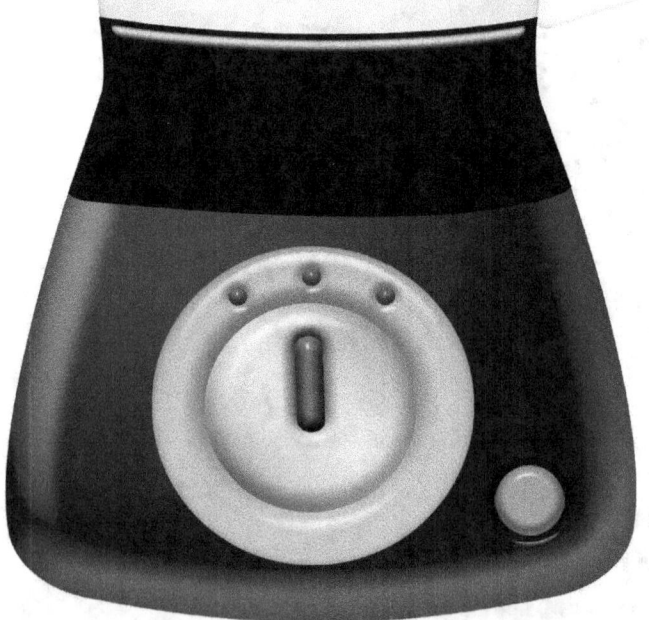

Juice to Feel Happy

1 Banana
½ Cup 1% Chocolate Milk
4 tbsp Peanut Butter
½ tsp Vanilla Extract
½ Dark Chocolate Bar
1 tbsp Whey Protein
2 tbsp Unsweetend Cocoa
1 tbsp Açaí Pulp

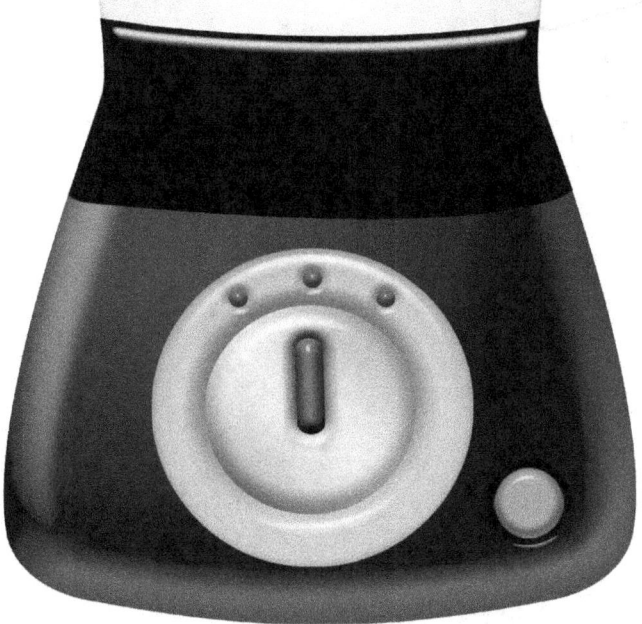

Juice for General Health

1 Banana, Sliced
¾ Cups of Vanilla Yogurt
1 tbsp Honey
½ tsp Freshly Grated Ginger
1 tsp Chia Seeds
1 Cup of Strawberries
Squeeze of Lemon

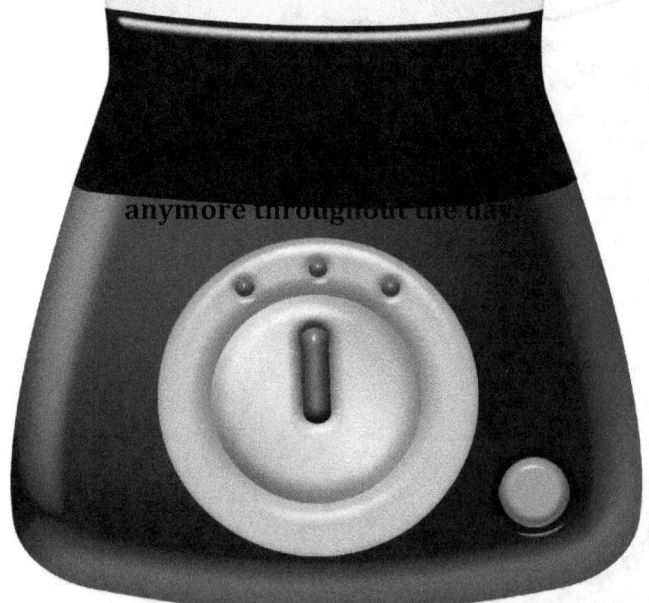

Juice for Kid's Health

- 1 ¼ Cup of Orange Juice
- ½ Avocado
- ¾ Cup Cranberries
- ½ Cup of Strawberries
- 1 Kiwi, Peeled
- 1 Frozen Banana
- 1 Cup Strawberry Yogurt
- 1 Children's Multivitamin

anymore throughout the day.

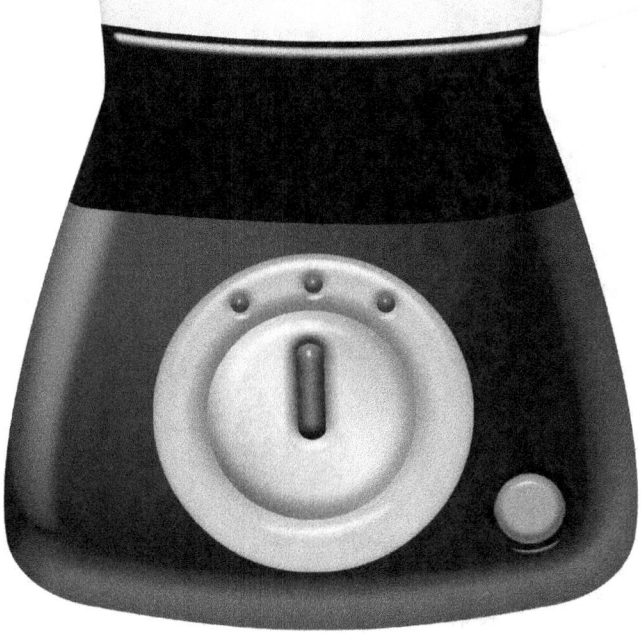

Juice for Senior's Health

8 oz Nutritional Shake, Vanilla
1 Cup of Ice Cubes
1 Cup of Yogurt, Strawberry
½ Cup Strawberries
½ Cup of Spinach
2 tbsp Granola
1 tbsp Oats, Raw

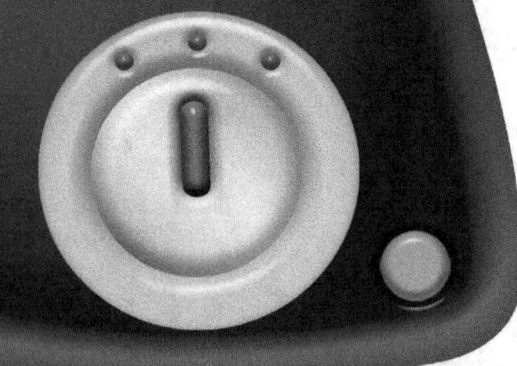

Juice For Healthy Heart

1½ Cup Cranberry Juice
1 tbsp Flaxseed Powder
1 tsp Chia Seed
1 tsp Honey
½ Cup Watermelon
1 tsp of Lemon Juice
1 Green Apple

* Please consult your doctor
Especially if you have heart
conditions before drinking.

Juice Lower Heart Disease

1 Banana
1 Orange
¼ Cup of Strawberries
¼ Cup of Raspberries
¼ Avocado
2 Cups of Spinach
1 tbsp Flaxseed Powder
2 tsp of Pumpkin Seeds
8 oz Almond Milk

* Please consult your doctor
  especially if you have heart
  conditions before drinking.

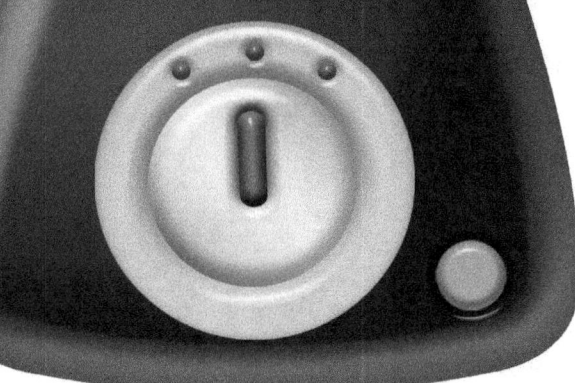

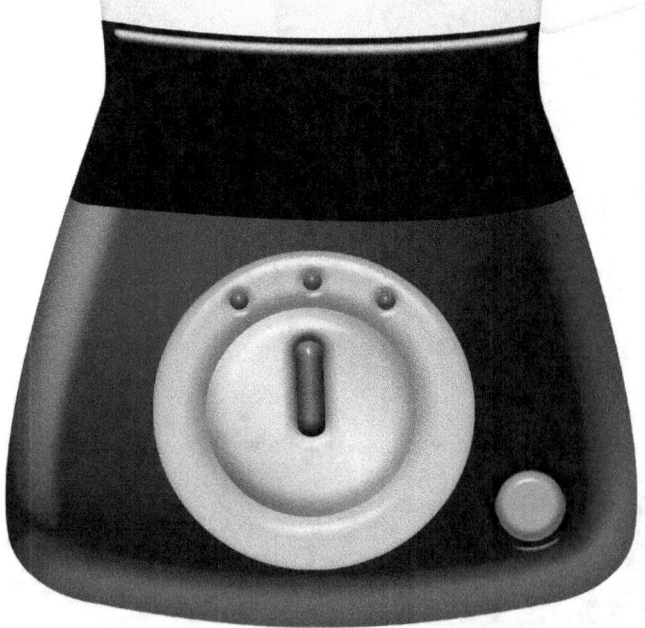

Juice for Hemorrhoids

1 Cup of cranberries
1 Green Pear
1 Cup of Ice Cubes
1 ½ Cup Greek Yogurt
2 tbsp Flaxseed
1 tsp of Ginger Root
2 Pitted Prunes

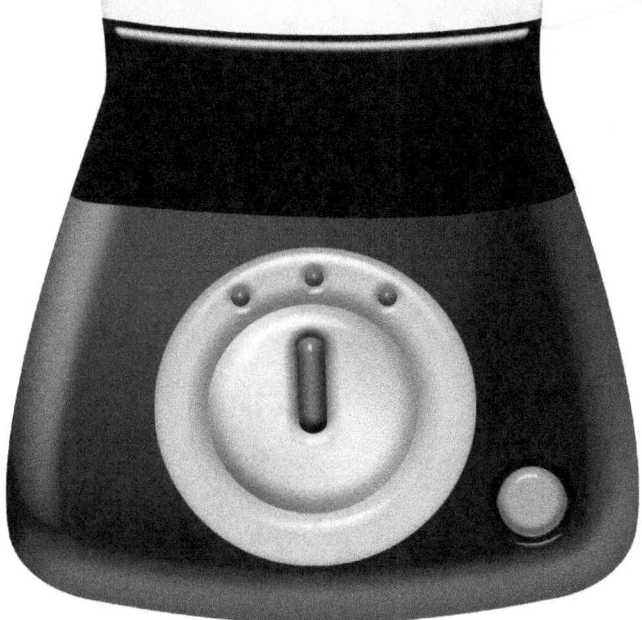

Juice for Hepatitis

1 tsp Choline Bitartrate, Powder
4 tbsp Strawberry Yogurt
4 Pineapple Slices
1 Mango
1 Apples
1 Lemon Squeezed
1 tbsp Ginger
2 tbsp Brown Rice
2 tbsp Quinoa

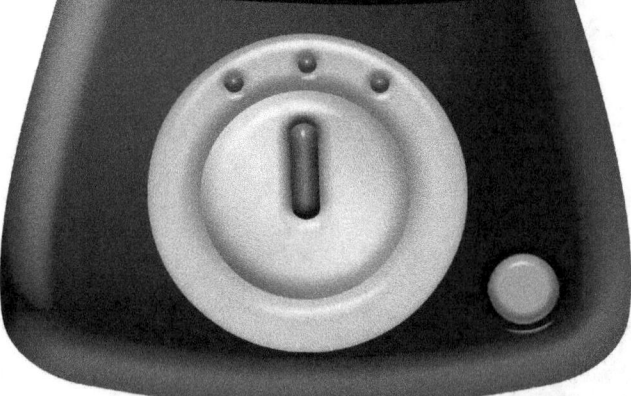

Juice to Fight off Herpes

1 Cup Greek Yogurt, Vanilla
1/3 Cup of Coconut, Shredded
½ Cup of Papaya
1 Apple, Green
1 Guava, Cubed
1 Cup of Milk
500 mg Capsule of lysine

Avoid eating peanuts,
chocolate, raisins, oatmeal and
caffeine. Consult your doctor.

Juice for Insomnia

1 Cup Cherries, Pitted
½ Banana
1 Cup Chamomile Tea
2 tbsp Soy Milk
 Pinch of nutmeg

* Serve warm.

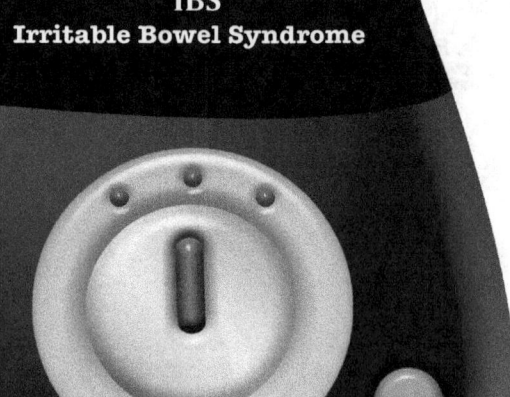

Juice for IBS

1 Cup Apple Cider
1 Pear, Sliced
1 Cup of Yogurt, Active Cultures
1 tbsp of Almond Butter
 Pinch of Cinnamon
 Pinch of Nutmeg

IBS
Irritable Bowel Syndrome

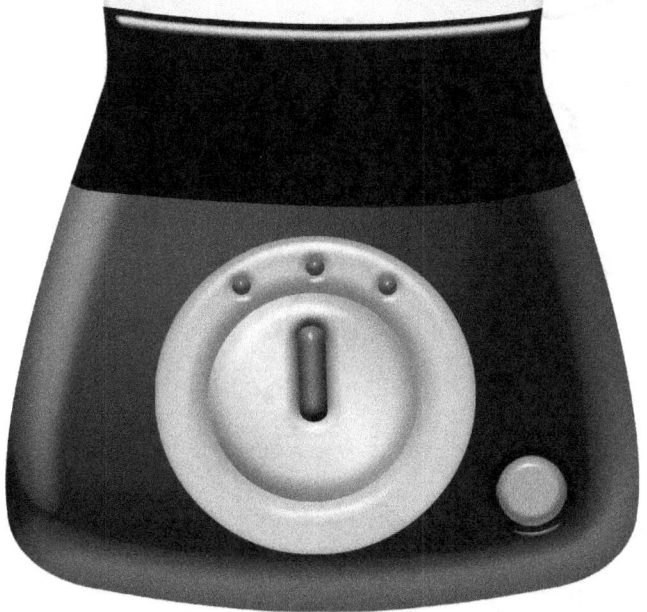

Juice for Jet Lag

3 tbsp of Hemp Seeds
1 Cup of Apple Juice
1 Banana, Frozen
½ Cup of Cherries, Frozen
Pinch of Vanilla Extract

Hemp (Cannabis sativa) is not psychoactive; so it is impossible get high by eating or drinking in Protein Powder hemp. Just understand that Hemp is not the same or associated with the drug cannabis.

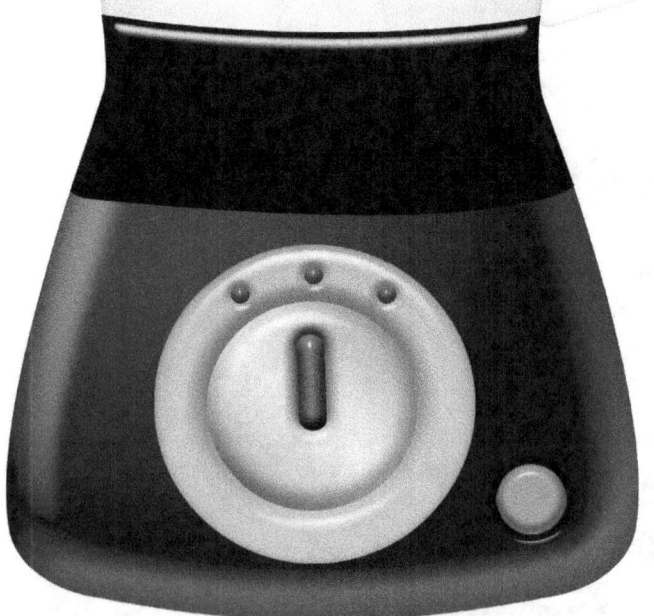

Juice for Lupus

6oz Yogurt, Vanilla
½ Cup of Orange Juice
1 Pineapple Slice
½ Mango, Remove Seed
3 Strawberries
1 Orange
½ Cup of Spinach
½ Cup of Kale
Handful of Ice Cubes
½ Banana

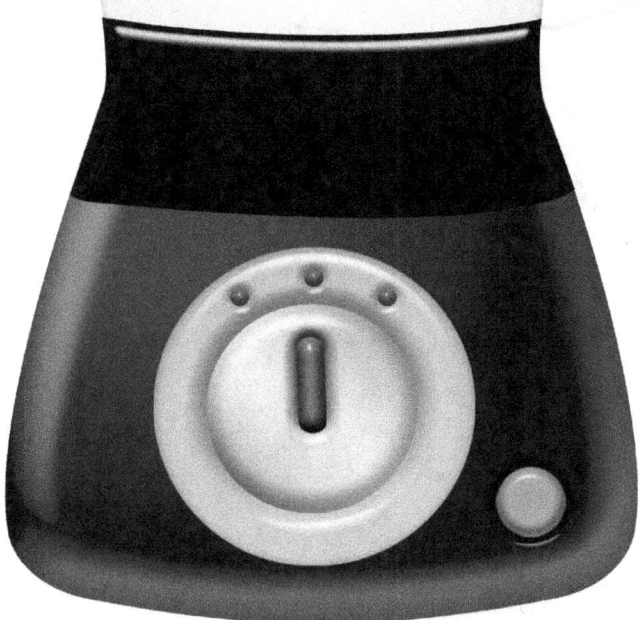

Juice for Menopause

½ Cup of Chickpeas (Isoflavones)
1 tbsp of Flaxseeds
½ tsp Ginseng Powder
1 Banana
1 Cup Kale
2 Kiwis, Peeled
1 Cup Soy Milk
½ tbsp Fiber
1 tsp Cinnamon
1 Vanilla Yogurt

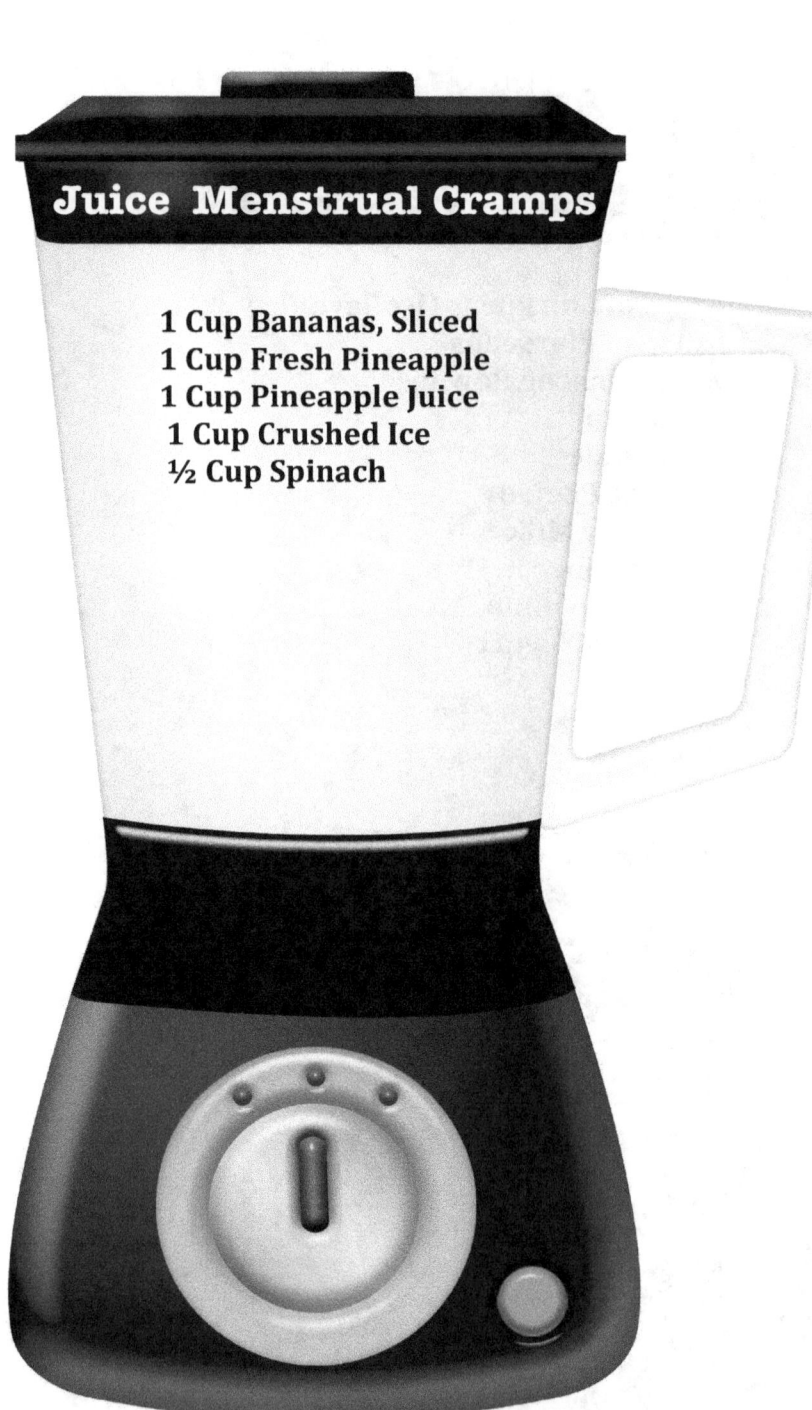

Juice Menstrual Cramps

1 Cup Bananas, Sliced
1 Cup Fresh Pineapple
1 Cup Pineapple Juice
1 Cup Crushed Ice
½ Cup Spinach

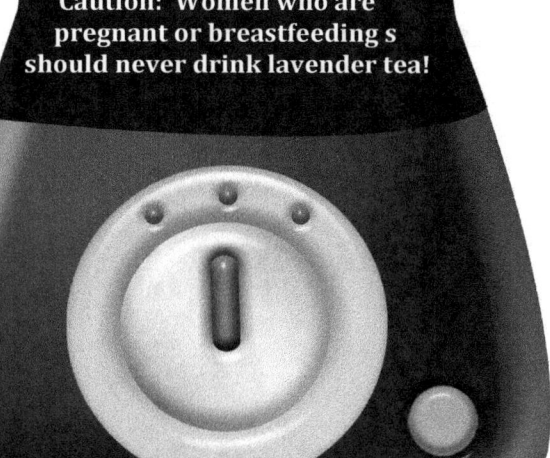

Juice for Migraines

½ Cup Lavender Tea
2/3 Yogurt, Lime
6 Strawberries
½ Cup Raspberries
1 tbsp Molasses
1 tsp Hemp Seeds
Pinch of Ginger
1 tbsp Coffee, Ground

Caution: Women who are
pregnant or breastfeeding s
should never drink lavender tea!

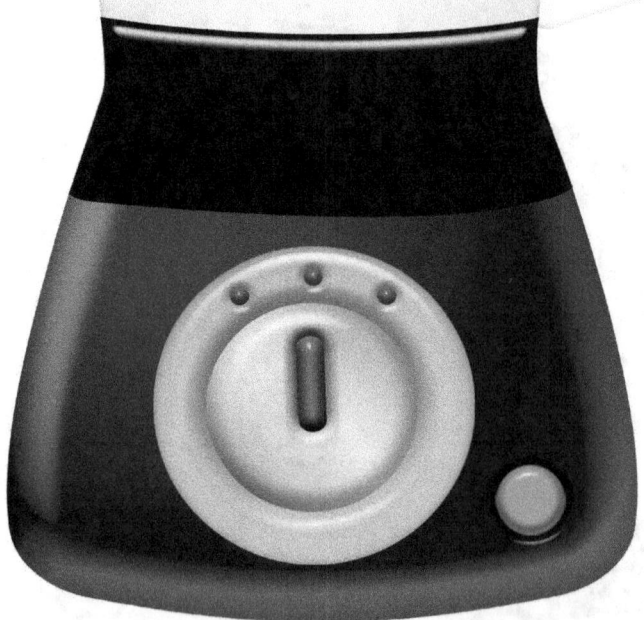

Juice for Muscle Building

½ Cup Yogurt, Chocolate
2 tbsp Peanut Butter
1 Frozen Banana
1/3 Cups of Whey Protein
1 Cup Chocolate Milk

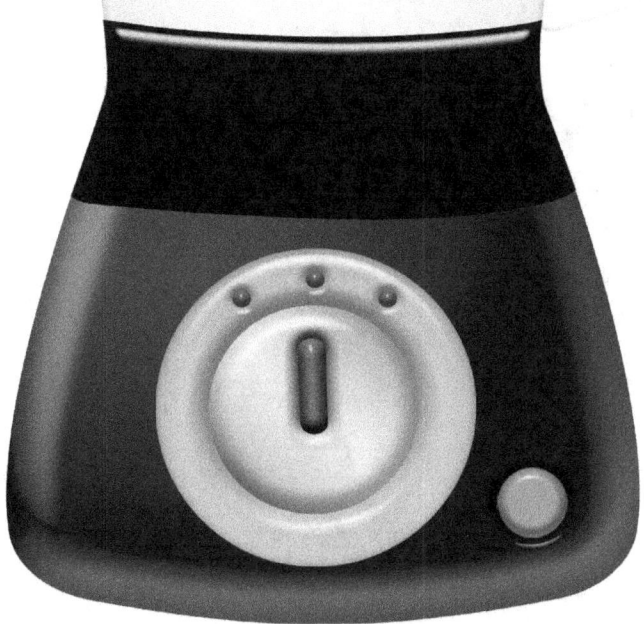

Juice for Muscle Pain

1 Celery Stalk
1 Banana
1 Cup of Cucumber, Sliced
1 Lemon, Squeezed
Pinch of Ginger
1 Cup of Coconut Water

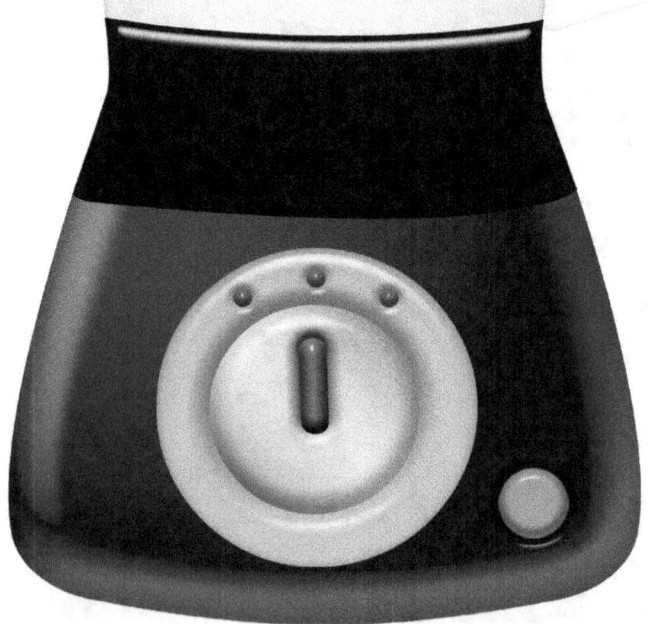

Juice for Nausea

1 Kiwi, Peeled
1 Cup Strawberries
2 Bananas
3 Mint Leaves
½ Greek yogurt
1 Inch Ginger Root
1 Cup of Coconut Water
1 Cup Ice Cubes

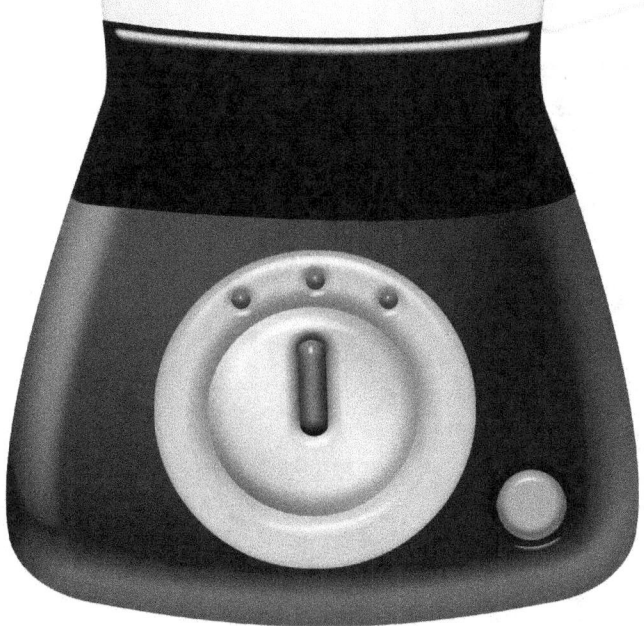

Juice Fight Obesity

1 Cup Mango Chunks
½ Avocado
1 Cup Green Tea
1 Cup Kale
½ tbsp Virgin Coconut Oil
2 Drops Agave
1 tsp Chia Seed

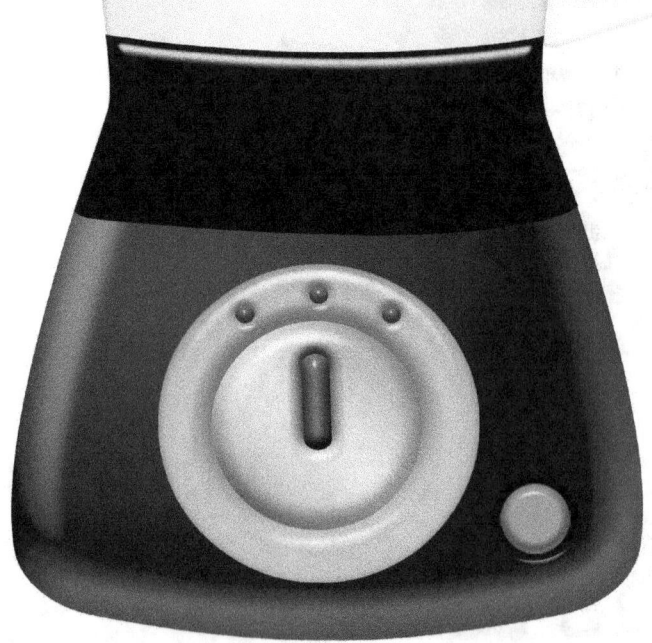

Juice for Osteoporosis

½ Cup Orange Juice with Calcium
1 ¼ Cup Mixed Berries
¾ Cup Yogurt, Vanilla
2 tbsp Powder Milk
1 tbsp Wheat Germ
1 tbsp Honey
½ tsp Vanilla Extract

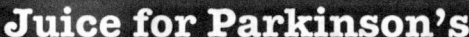

Juice for Parkinson's

2 Cups of Almond Milk
2 Frozen Bananas
1 tbsp of Cashews
1 tbsp of Walnuts
1 tbsp of Pistachio
1 tbsp Peanuts, Unsalted
2 Cups Vanilla Yogurt

Men and women who consumed a
diet rich in anthocyanins (antioxidants)
had a lower risk of Parkinson's disease

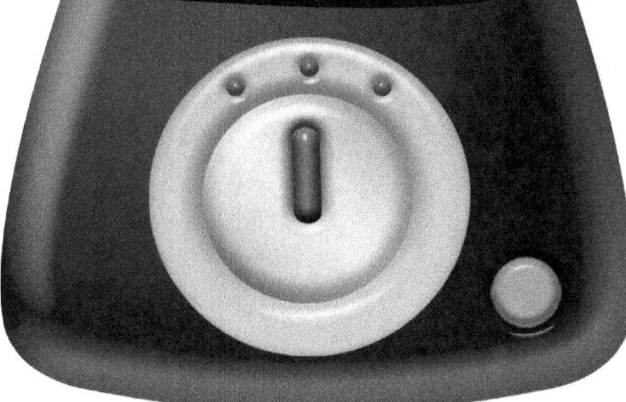

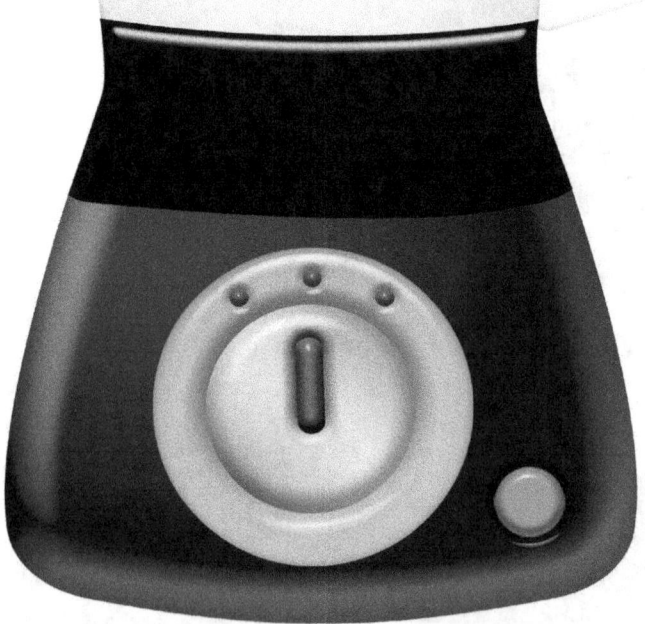

Juice for Attraction

1 Cup Dark Chocolate
1 tsp Chili Powder
1 ½ Cup Almond Milk
1 tbsp Honey
2 tsp Granola
½ Cup Raspberries
1 Celery Stalk

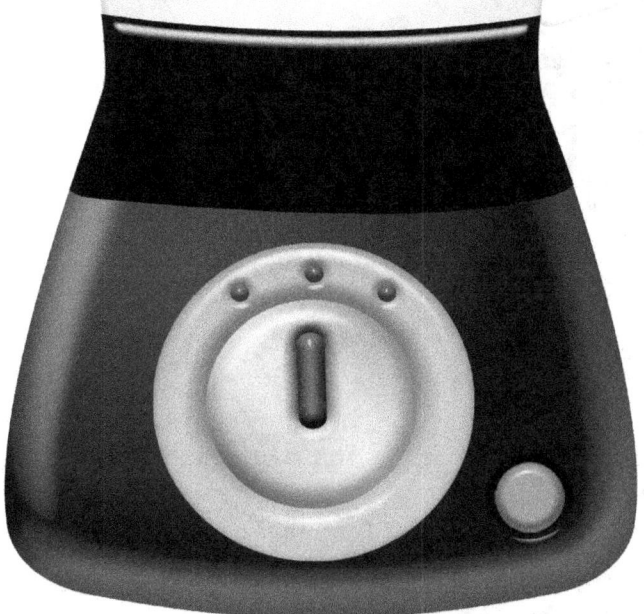

Juice for Healthy Pregnancy

1 cup of spinach
½ tbsp Flax Hemp Blend
1 ½ Cup Organic Berries
1 Organic Banana
1 cup almond milk
1 cup yogurt, Strawberry
½ tbsp cacao, powder
½ tbsp Coconut Oil

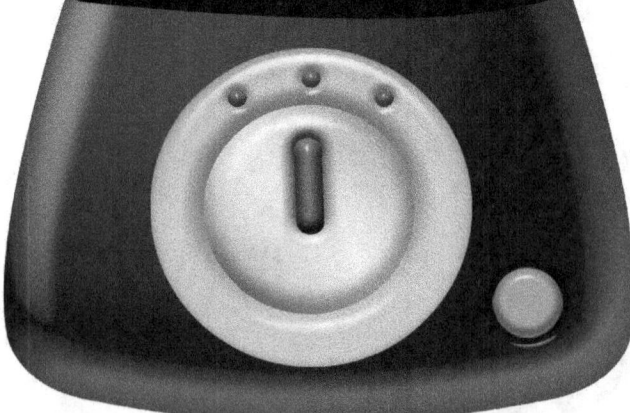

Juice for Sexual Pleasure

12 oz Low Fat Milk
½ tsp Zinc Sulfate
1 tsp Ginger
12 Drops of Ginseng
1 Drop of Selenium
4 Strawberries
½ Banana, Peeled

* Consult your doctor first

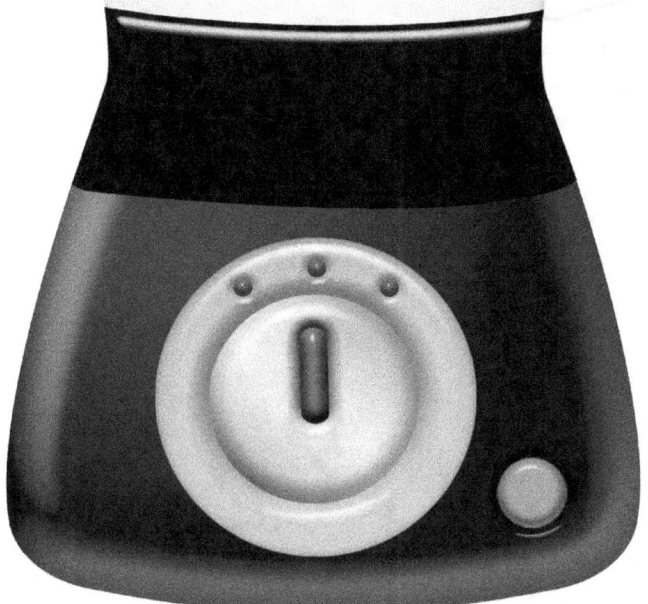

Juice Help Psoriasis

1 Cup Green Tea
1/3 Medium Avocado
1 Kiwi, skin Peeled
1 Cup Baby Spinach
1/2 Cup Frozen Blueberries
1 tbsp Chia Seeds
1/2 tsp Turmeric
1/2 tsp Ginger
½ tsp Cinnamon
½ tsp Turmeric

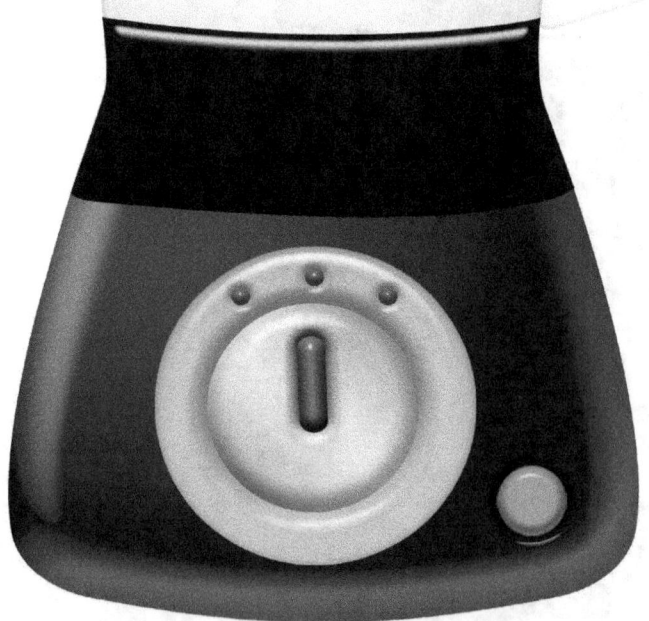

Juice for Puberty

1 Can of Pumpkin
1 Can Coconut Milk
1 Pear, Cored
½ Cup Pecans
1 tsp Flaxseed Powder
1 tbsp Cinnamon
Pinch of Cardamom
2 tsp Vanilla Extract

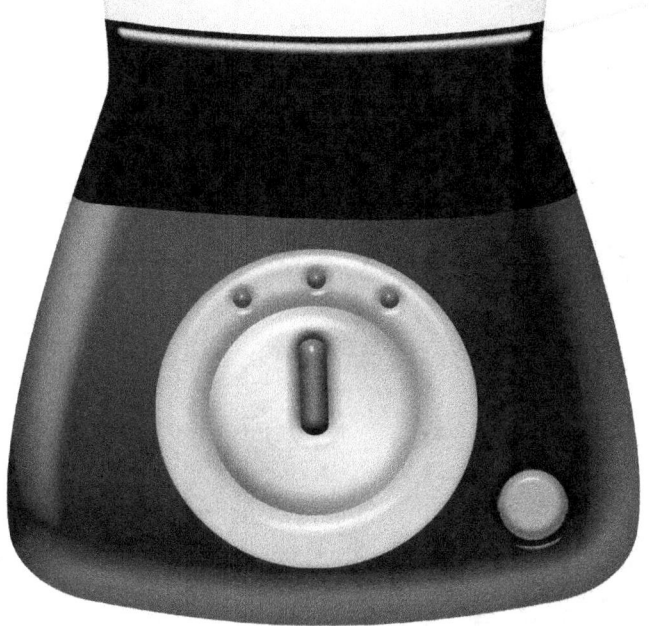

Juice for Smoking

1 tbsp Seaweed Powder
1 Cup Rice Bran
1 tsp Pumpkin Seeds
1 tsp Sunflower Seeds
1 tsp Flaxseeds
1 tsp Mint
1 Cup Yogurt, Chocolate
4 Pieces Dark Chocolate
½ Cup Almond Milk

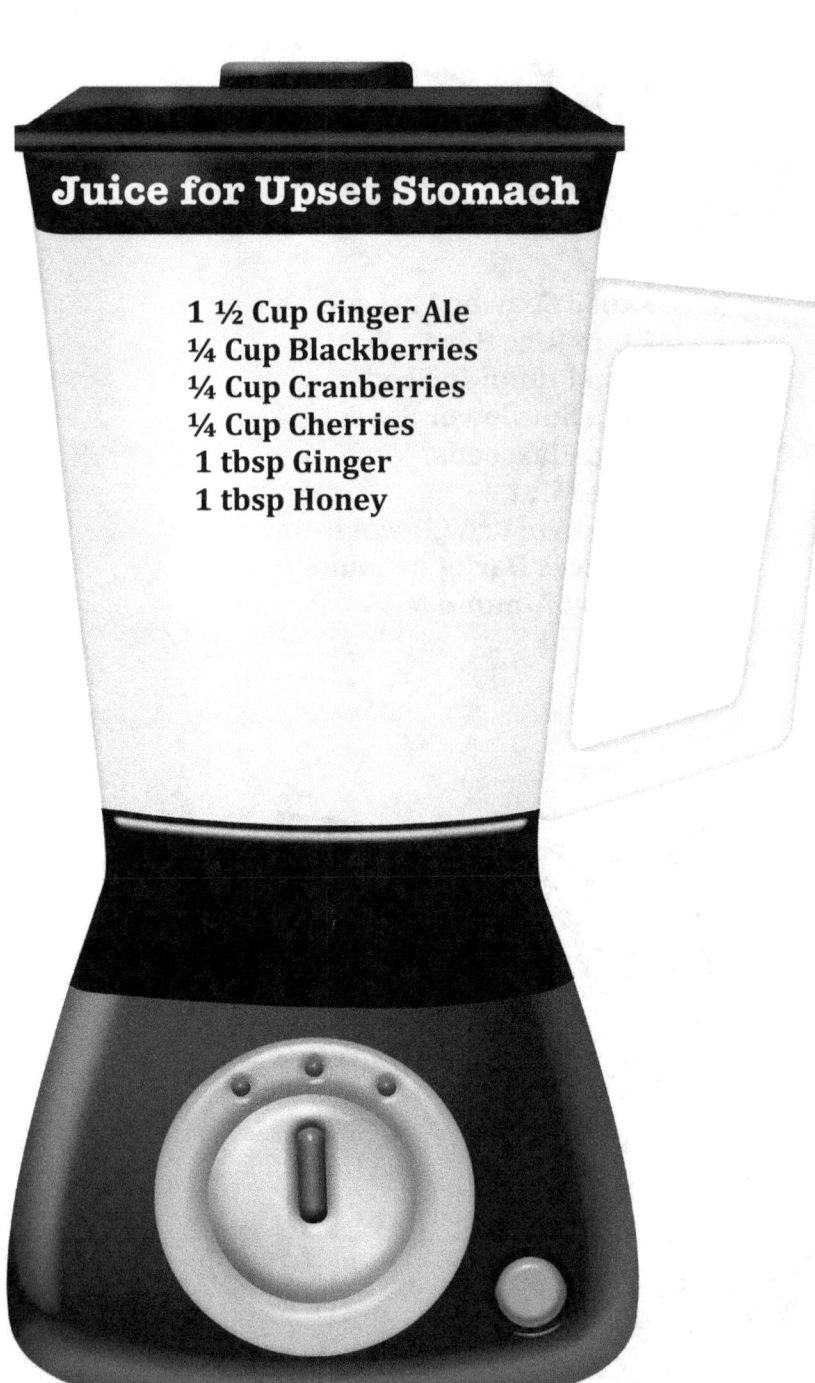

Juice for Upset Stomach

1 ½ Cup Ginger Ale
¼ Cup Blackberries
¼ Cup Cranberries
¼ Cup Cherries
1 tbsp Ginger
1 tbsp Honey

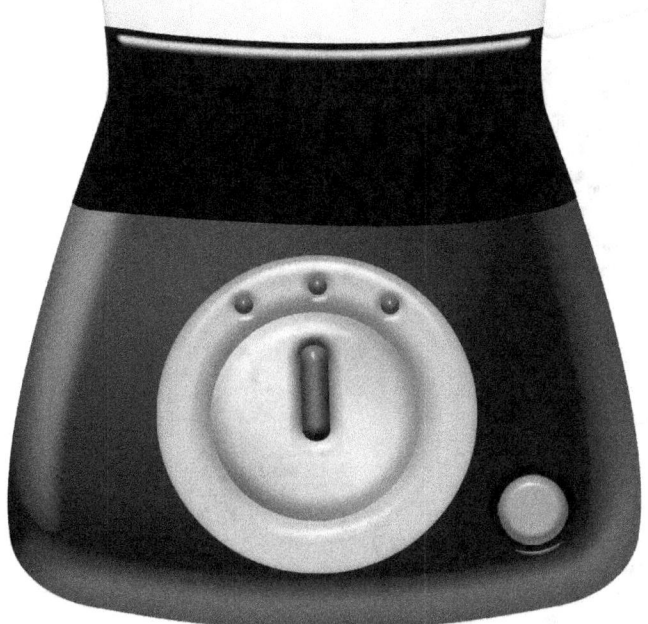

Juice for Flatter Tummy

1 tbsp Whey Protein, Vanilla
1 Yogurt, Low Fat
¼ Cup Berries
¼ Cup Raspberries
¼ Cup Strawberries
½ Cup Low Fat Milk
3 Ice Cubes

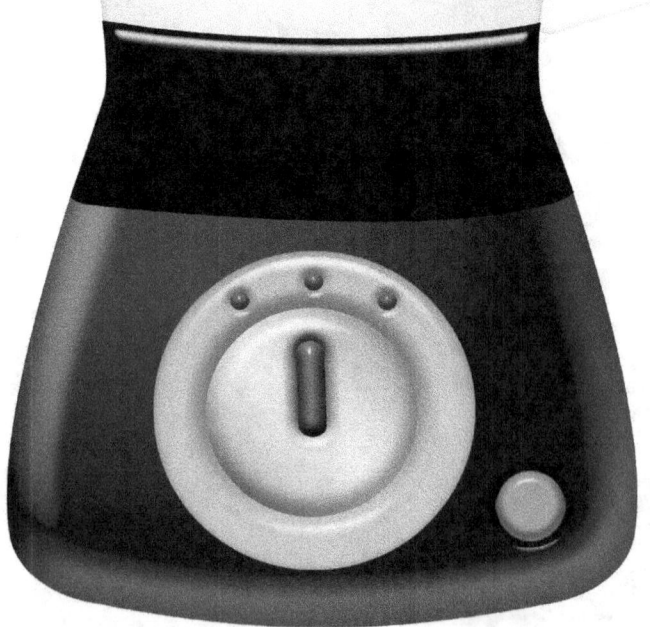

Juice for Stress

2 Celery Stalks
2 tbsp Fennel
1 Cup Lettuce
1 Cup of Pineapple
1 tbsp Agave
1 tsp Chia Powder
½ Cup Pineapple Juice
1 tsp Cinnamon

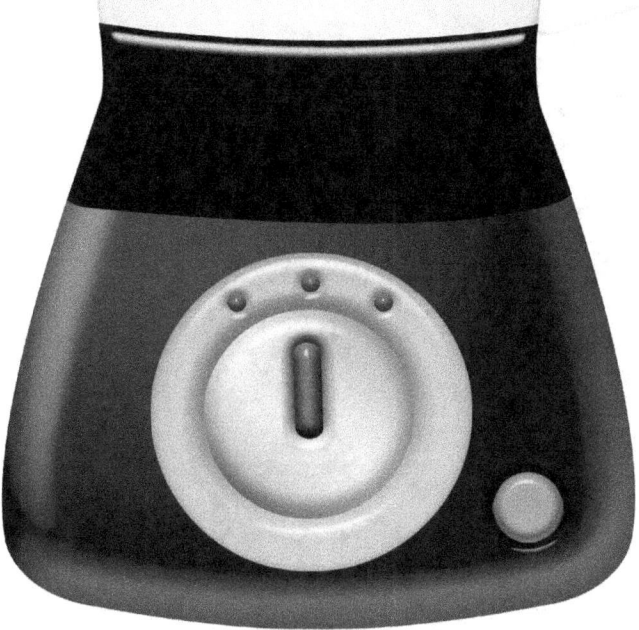

Juice Help Reduce Stroke

3 Cabbage Leaves
1 Cup of Kale
1 Beet
½ tsp Dried Basil
1 ½ Cup Low Fat Yogurt
2 Tomatoes, Peeled
2 tbsp Pumpkin Seeds
1 tbsp Cashews
Dash of Pepper

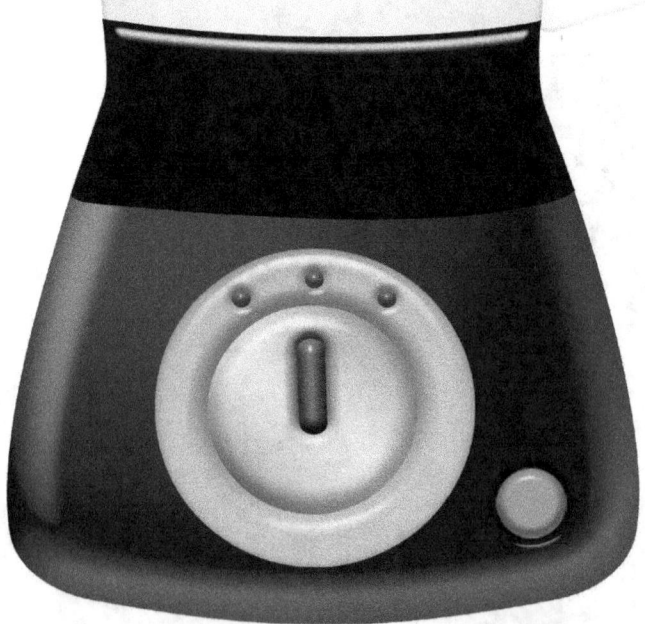

Juice for Sore Throat

2/3 Cups Cranberry Juice
1 Cup Raspberries
½ Inch Piece Ginger
1 Melon Slice
1 tsp Lemon
2 tsp Honey
Small Piece Aloe, Peeled

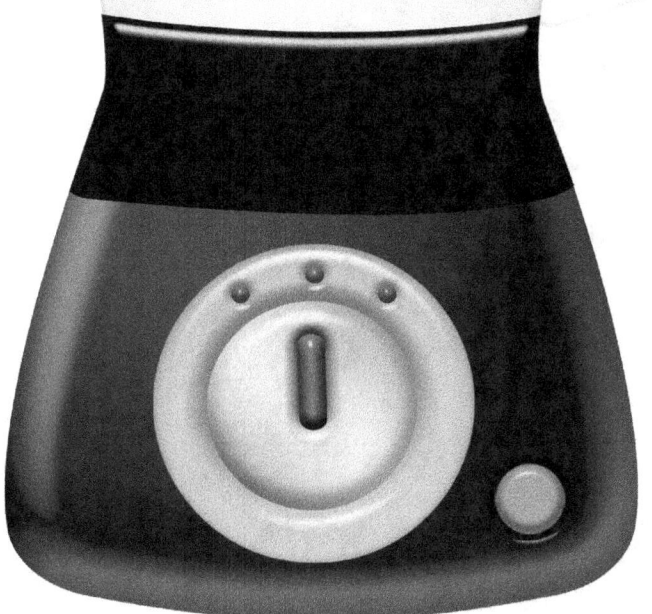

Juice for Thyroid

½ Banana
1 Cucumber
1 Cup Spinach
1 tbsp Honey
1 tbsp Hemp Seeds
1 tsp Matcha Powder
1 tsp Spirulina Powder
1 tbsp Coconut Butter
Dash of Cinnamon
2 Cups of Vanilla Yogurt

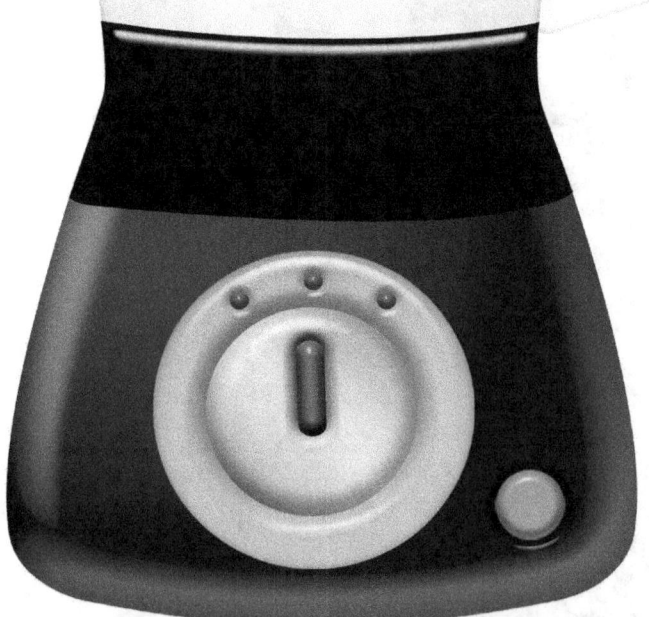

Juice for Ulcers

½ Diced Pineapple
Pinch of Ginger
1 Cup Chamomile Tea
2 Apples, Cored
2 tbsp Aloe vera Gel
6 Cabbage Leaves
1 Cup 100% Apple Juice

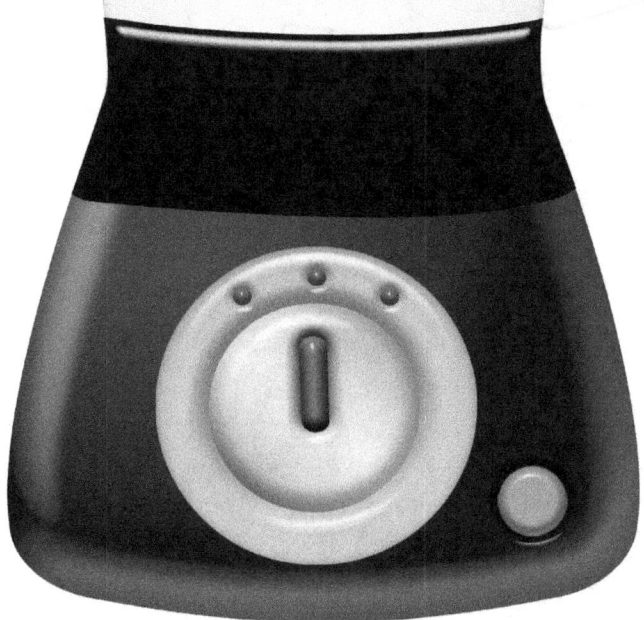

Juice for UTI

1 ½ Cup Cranberry Juice
½ Cup Raspberries
1 Cup Dry Cranberries
4 oz Yogurt, Vanilla
½ Cup Ice Cubes

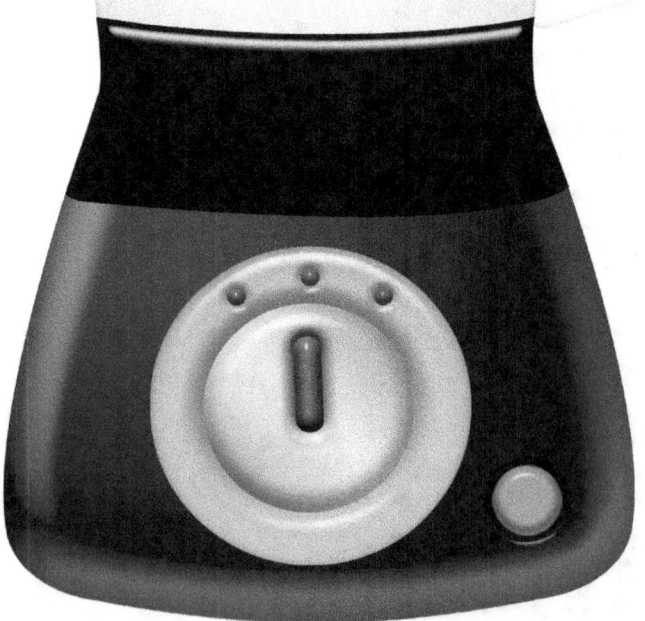

Juice for Varicose Veins

1 Cup White Grape Juice
1 Red Apple, Cored
½ Cup Blueberries
½ Cup of Beets
1 tsp Ginger
1 tsp Agave
½ Cup Coconut Milk
½ Cup Brown Rice

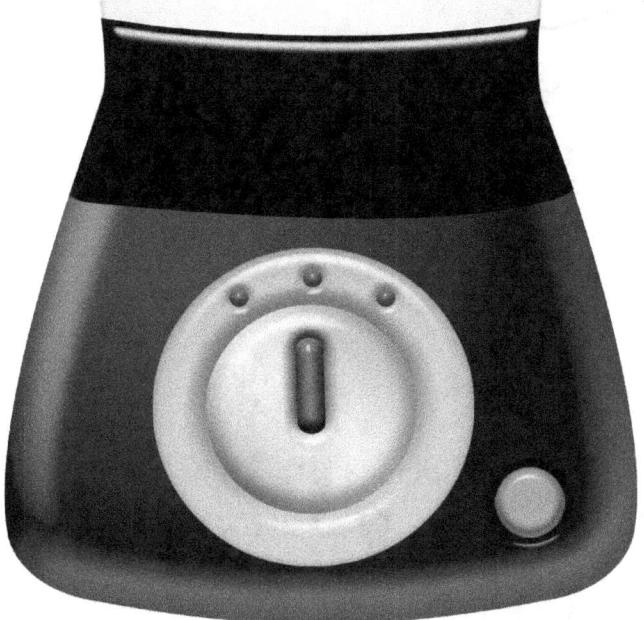

Juice for Vertigo

1 Frozen Banana
½ Kale Leaf
1 Cup Raspberries
4 Slices of Mango
½ Cup of Pomegranate
1 ½ Cups of coconut Water
2 tbsp Shredded Coconut

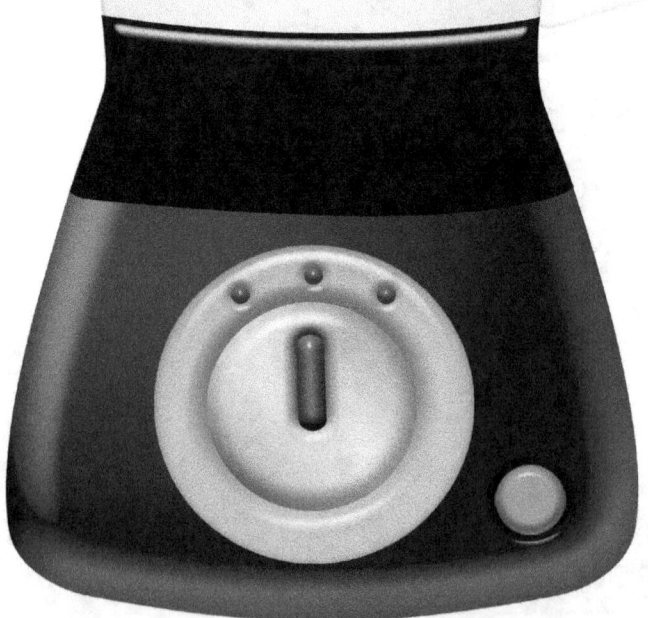

Juice Full of Vitamins

2 Oranges, Peeled
1 Peach, Cored
1 Banana
5 Strawberries
4 Cherries, Pitted
1/3 Cup Spinach
1 tbsp Walnuts
1 Cup Almond Milk
½ Cup Ice Cubes
1 tbsp Vanilla Extract

Juice to Whiten Teeth

½ Cup of Pineapple Chunks
1 Carrot, Chopped
1 tsp Ginger
1 tbsp Sunflower Seeds
2 Mushrooms
½ Apple, Cored
2 Basil Leaves
1 tsp Parsley, dried
5 Strawberries

Swish this smoothie around your mouth before swallowing since it contains properties such as malic acid that can help fight stains on your teeth.

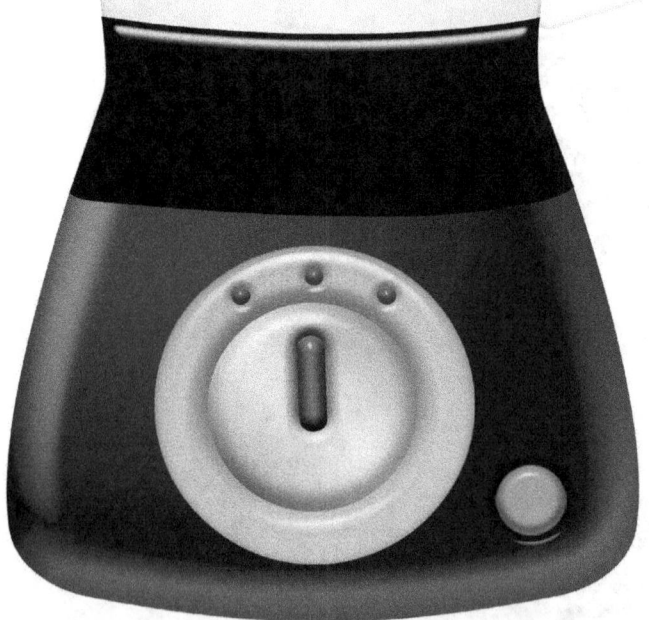

Juice Anti-Wrinkles

1 Cup Cranberry Juice
3 Cherries, Pitted
1 Cup of Mixed Berries
¼ Avocado
2 tbsp Wheat Germ
2 tbsp Flaxseed Powder
½ Cup Berry Yogurt
1 inch Aloe Gel
1 tbsb Unsalted Almonds

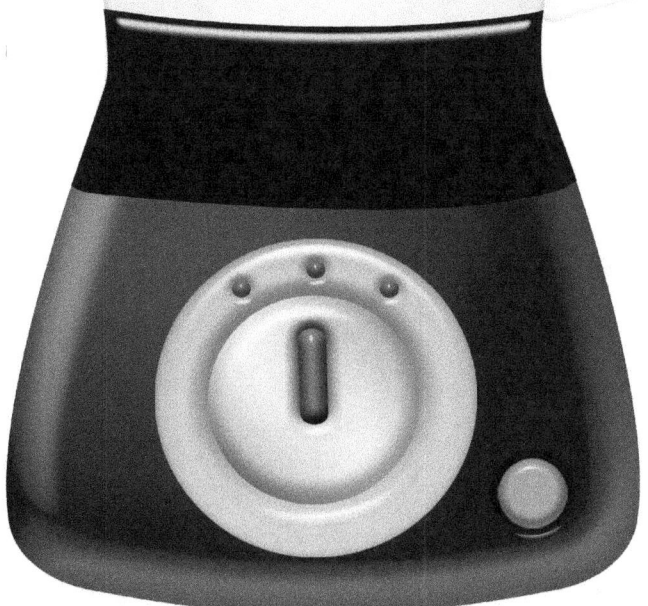

Juice for a Younger You

5 Romaine Lettuce Leaves
1 Cup of Baby Kale
5 Sprigs of Parsley
1/2 Large Lemon
1 Apple, Cored
1 Frozen Banana
1 tbsp Ground Flax Seeds
2 tbsp Ground Chia Seeds
1 Cup of Water
1/16 tsp of Honey
1/2 " Ginger
1/3 Cucumber, Sliced

Juicy Life
Desserts

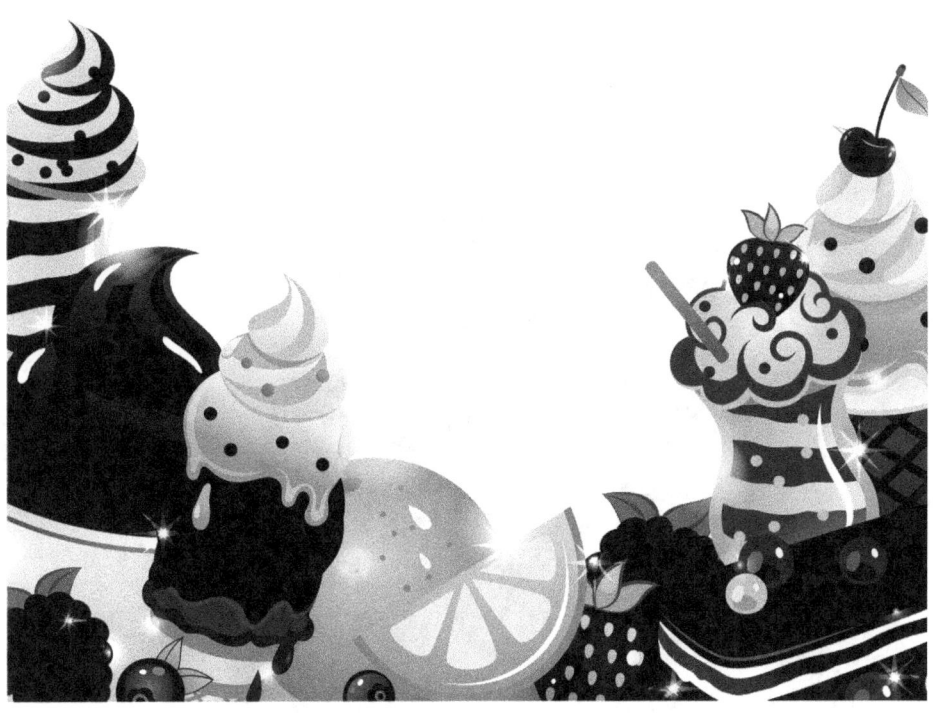

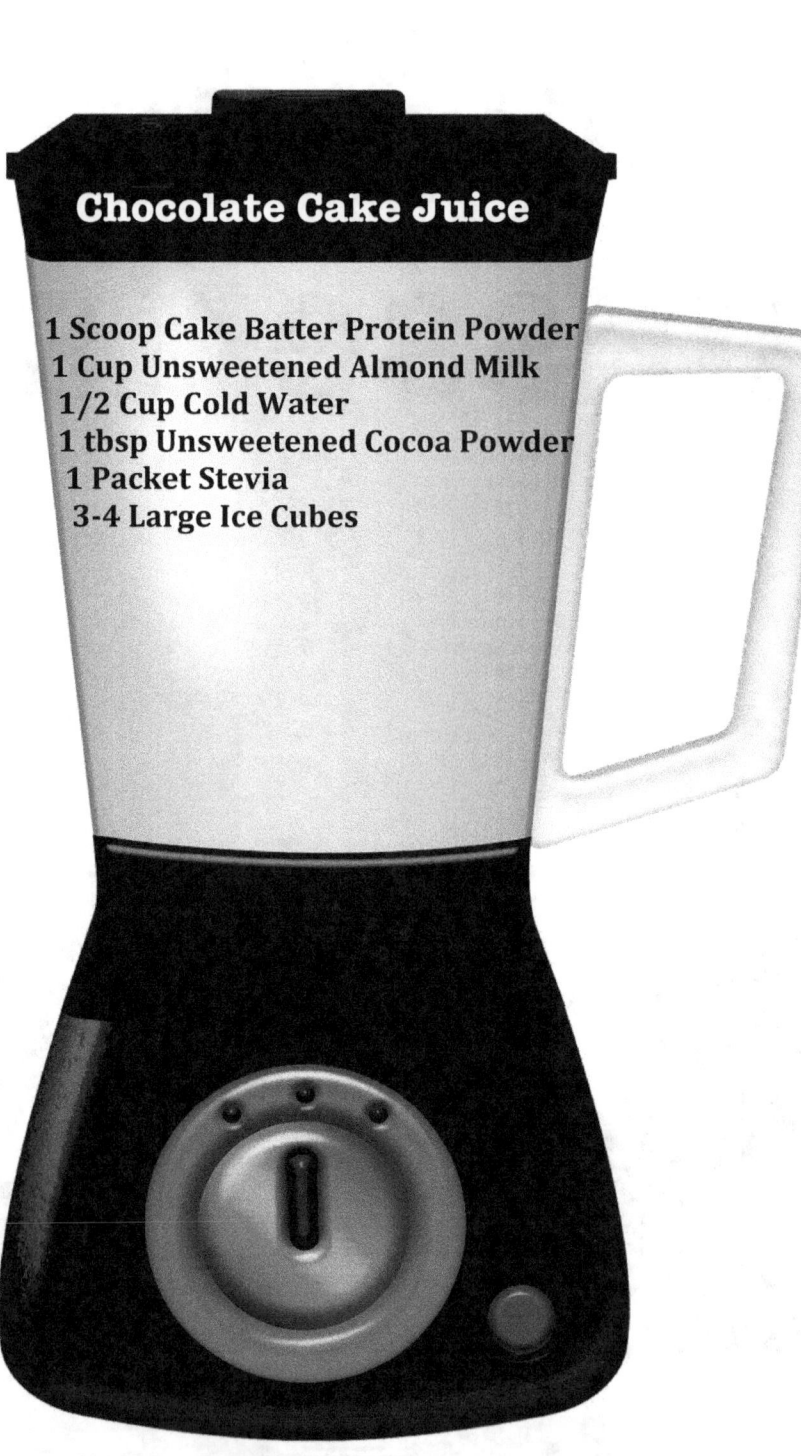

Chocolate Cake Juice

1 Scoop Cake Batter Protein Powder
1 Cup Unsweetened Almond Milk
1/2 Cup Cold Water
1 tbsp Unsweetened Cocoa Powder
1 Packet Stevia
3-4 Large Ice Cubes

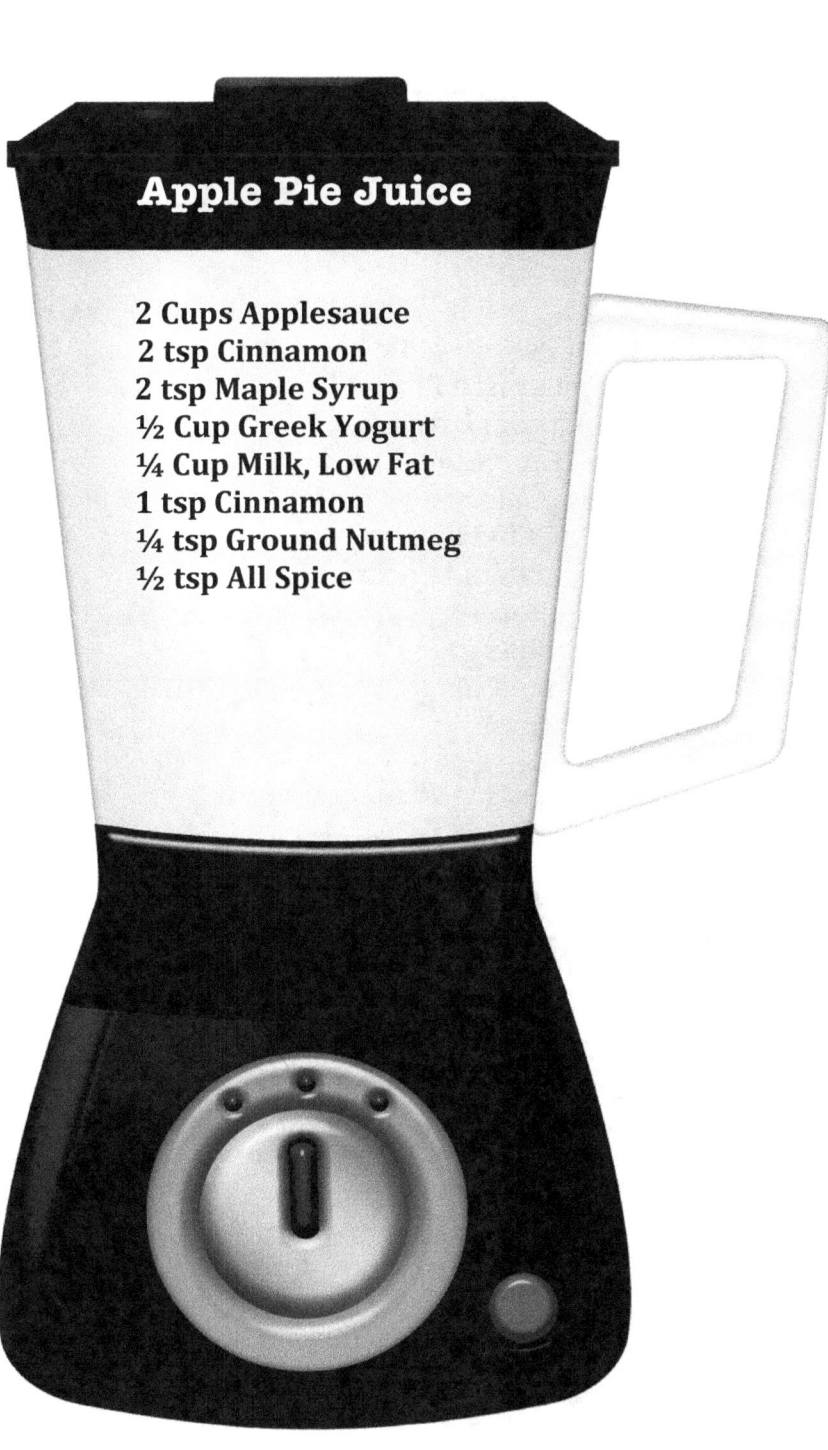

Apple Pie Juice

2 Cups Applesauce
2 tsp Cinnamon
2 tsp Maple Syrup
½ Cup Greek Yogurt
¼ Cup Milk, Low Fat
1 tsp Cinnamon
¼ tsp Ground Nutmeg
½ tsp All Spice

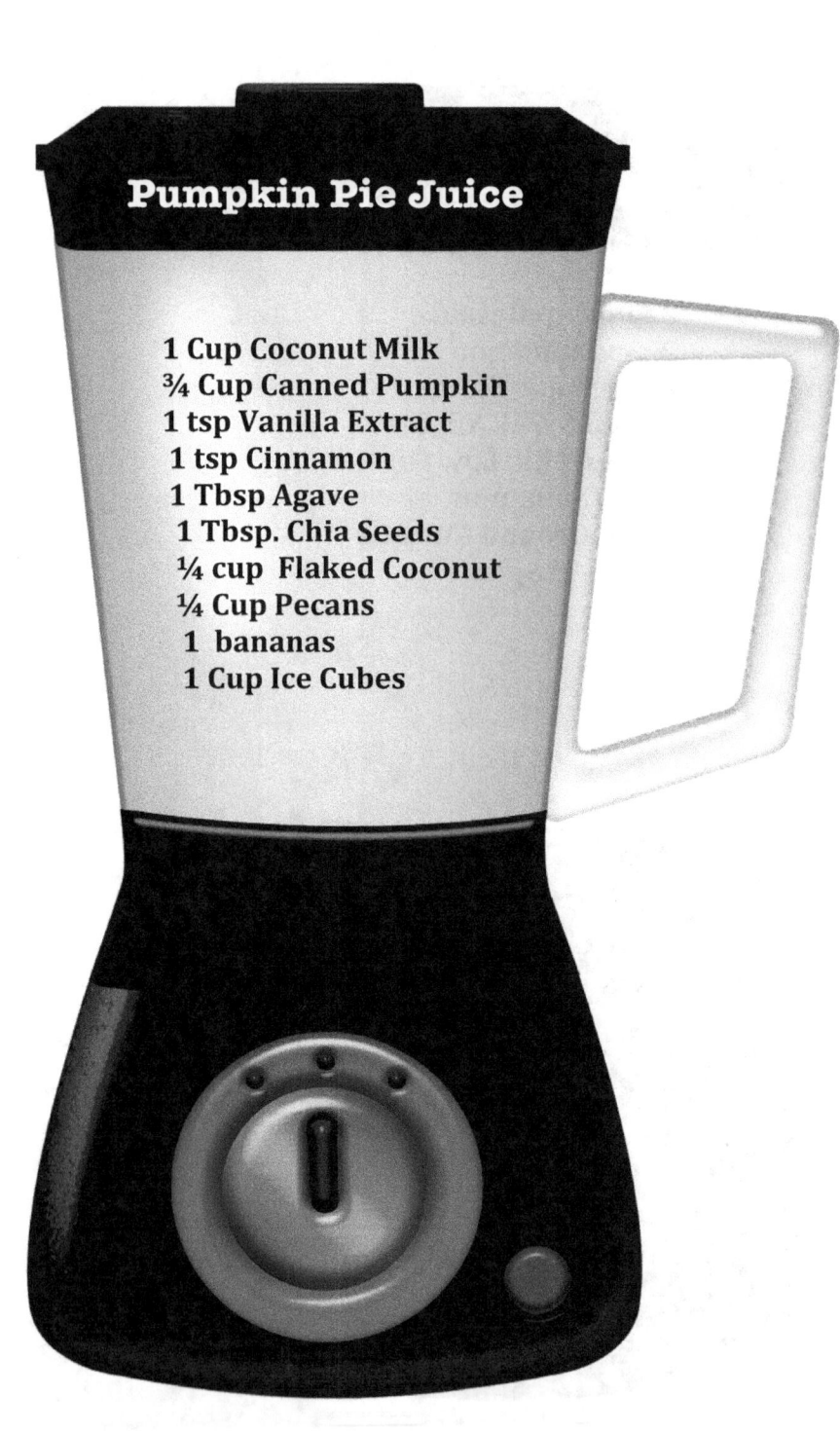

Pumpkin Pie Juice

1 Cup Coconut Milk
¾ Cup Canned Pumpkin
1 tsp Vanilla Extract
1 tsp Cinnamon
1 Tbsp Agave
1 Tbsp. Chia Seeds
¼ cup Flaked Coconut
¼ Cup Pecans
1 bananas
1 Cup Ice Cubes

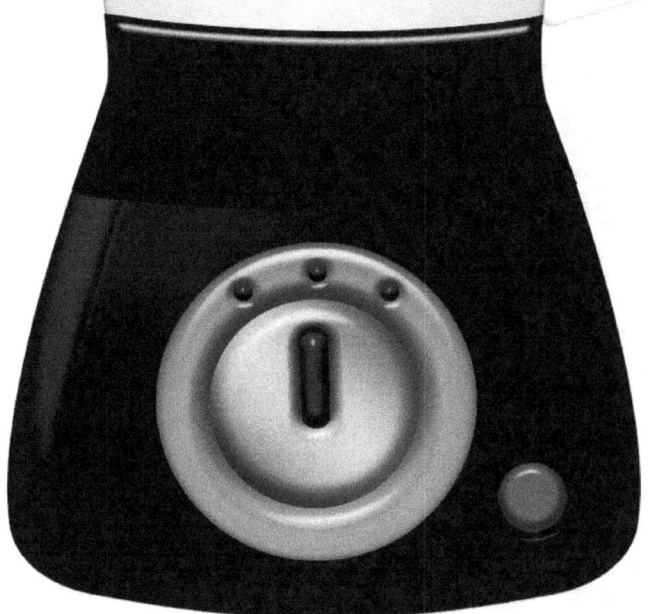

Red velvet Cake Juice

1/4 Cup Grated Beets
1/2 Cup Cottage Cheese
1 Scoop Chocolate Protein
1/3 Cup Rolled Oats
1/2 tsp Cinnamon
1/8 tsp Cake Batter Extract
1/2 Cup Milk
6 Ice Cubes
 Unsweetened Cocoa

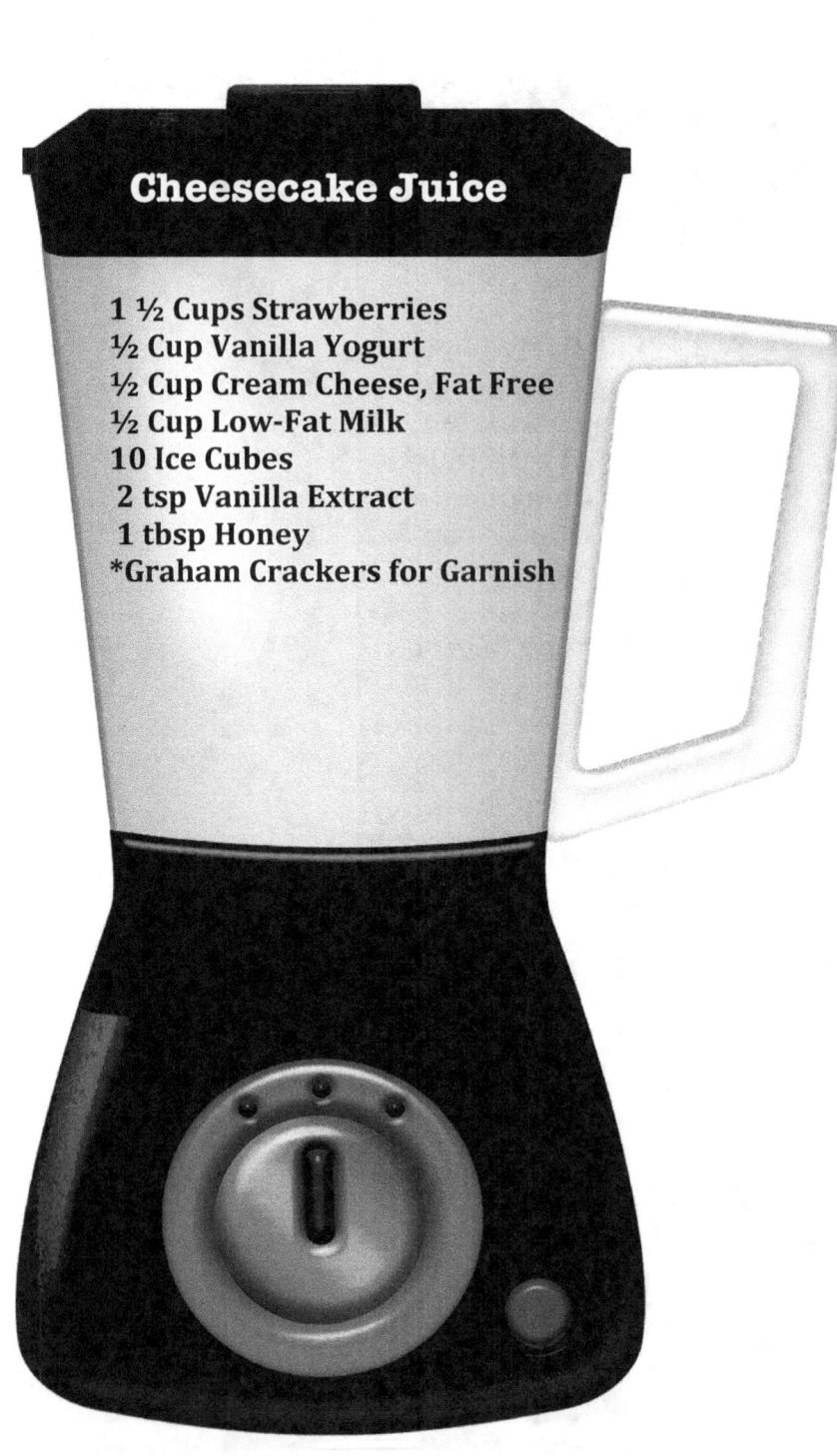

Cheesecake Juice

1 ½ Cups Strawberries
½ Cup Vanilla Yogurt
½ Cup Cream Cheese, Fat Free
½ Cup Low-Fat Milk
10 Ice Cubes
 2 tsp Vanilla Extract
 1 tbsp Honey
*Graham Crackers for Garnish

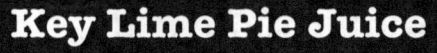

Key Lime Pie Juice

2 tbsp Key Lime Juice
1 tsp Key Lime Zest
1 Cup Unsweetened Milk
1 Banana
¼ tsp Vanilla Extract
2 Drops Stevia
1/2 tbsp Sunflower Butter
2 Cups Baby Spinach
4 Ice Cubes

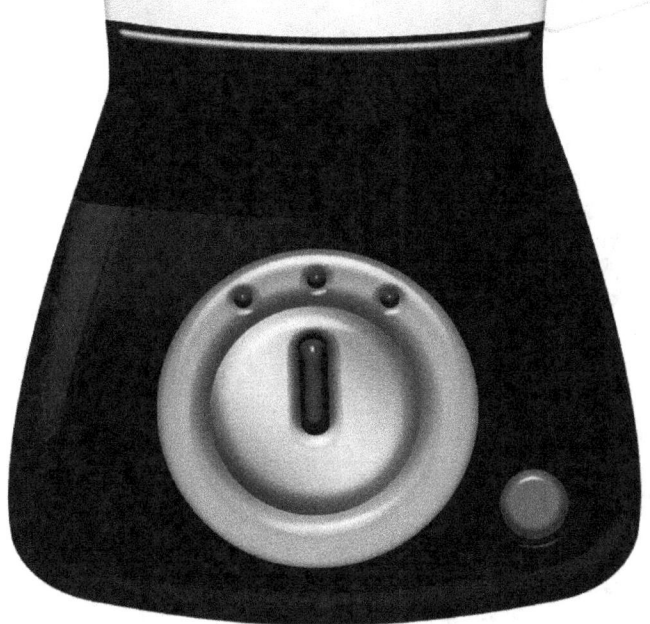

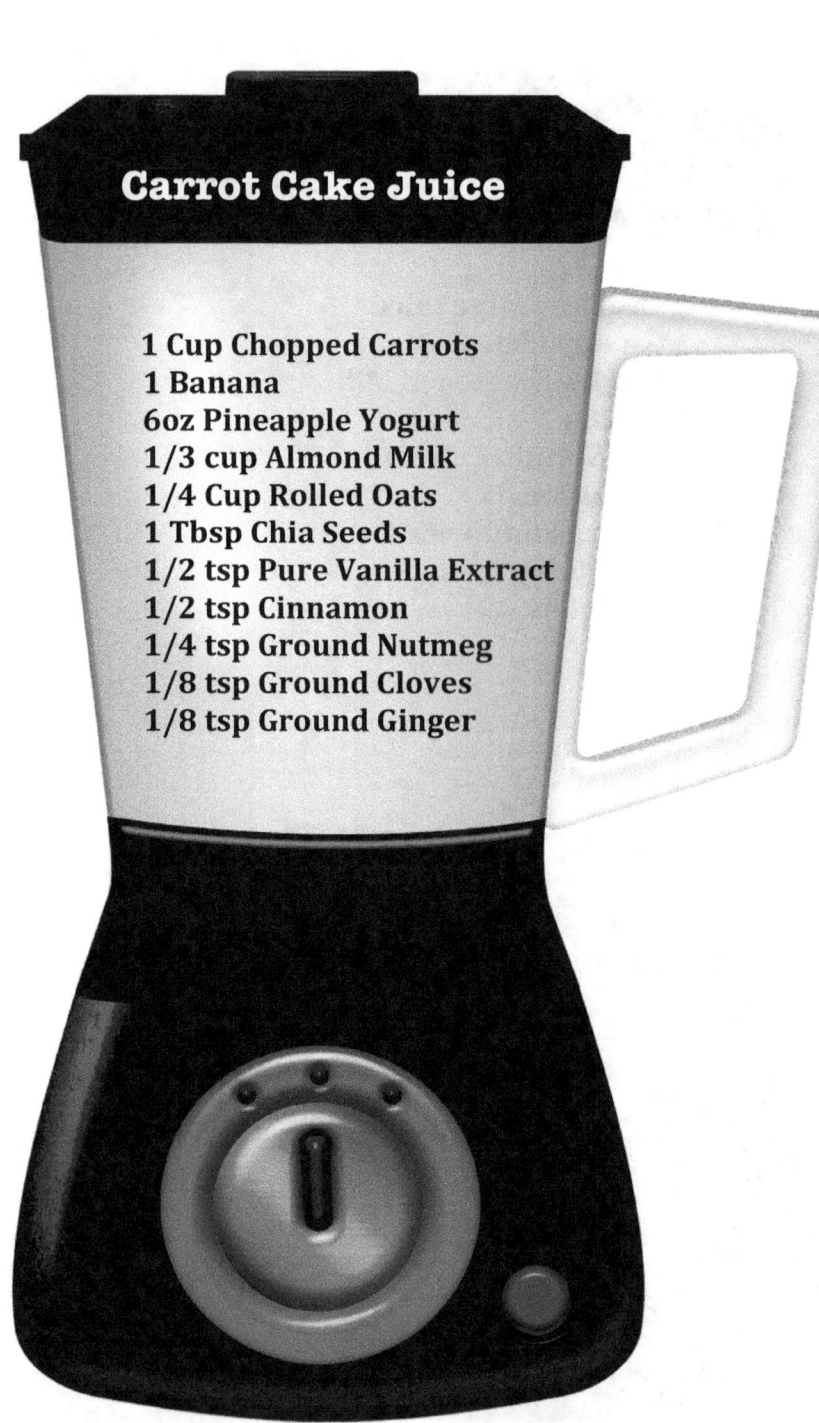

Carrot Cake Juice

1 Cup Chopped Carrots
1 Banana
6oz Pineapple Yogurt
1/3 cup Almond Milk
1/4 Cup Rolled Oats
1 Tbsp Chia Seeds
1/2 tsp Pure Vanilla Extract
1/2 tsp Cinnamon
1/4 tsp Ground Nutmeg
1/8 tsp Ground Cloves
1/8 tsp Ground Ginger

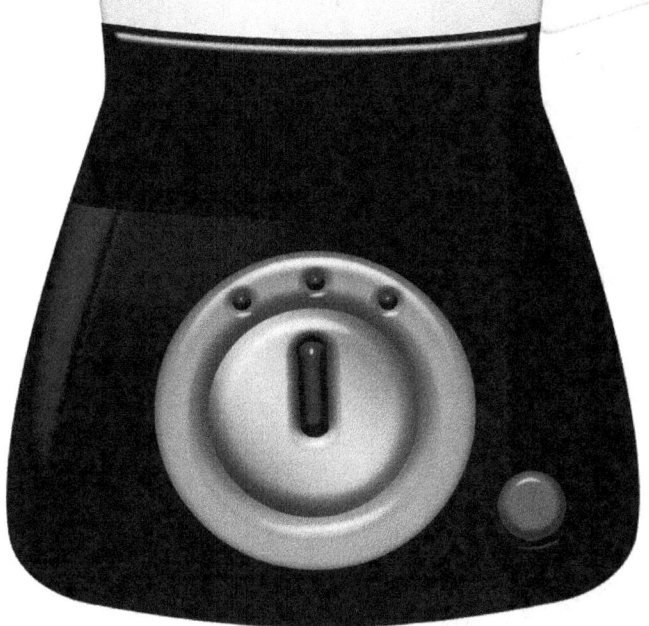

Banana Cream Pie Juice

- 1 Box of Instant Banana Pudding
- 1 Banana
- ½ tsp Cinnamon
- 1 tsp Vanilla Extract
- 2 tbsp Caramel Sauce Sugar Free
- 3 Cups Ice Cubes
- 1 tbsp Sugar
- 2 tbsp Peanut Butter
- 1 tbsp Butterscotch (Garnish)
- 1 tbsp White Chocolate Chips
- Caramel Sauce as Drizzle

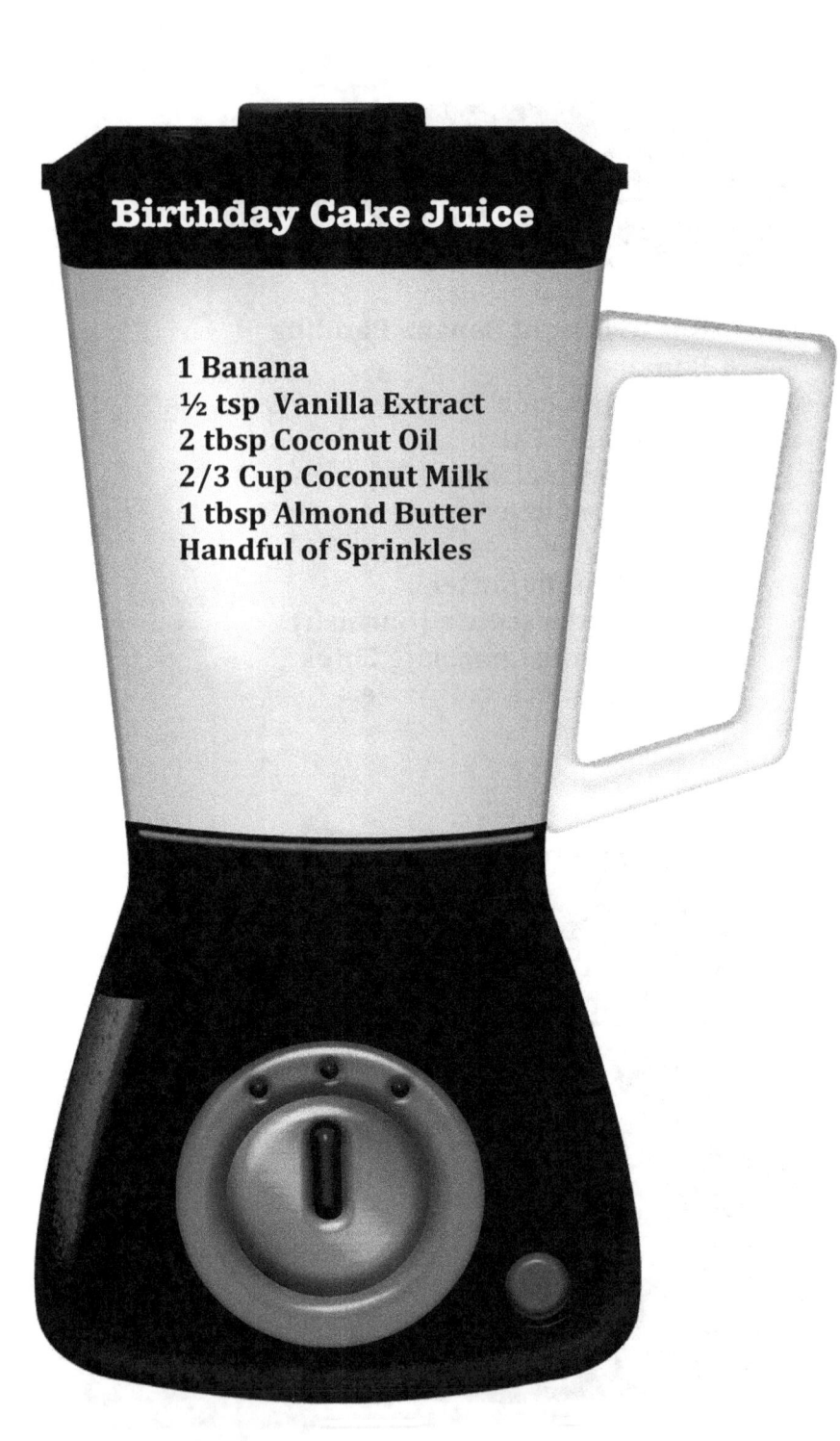

Birthday Cake Juice

1 Banana
½ tsp Vanilla Extract
2 tbsp Coconut Oil
2/3 Cup Coconut Milk
1 tbsp Almond Butter
Handful of Sprinkles

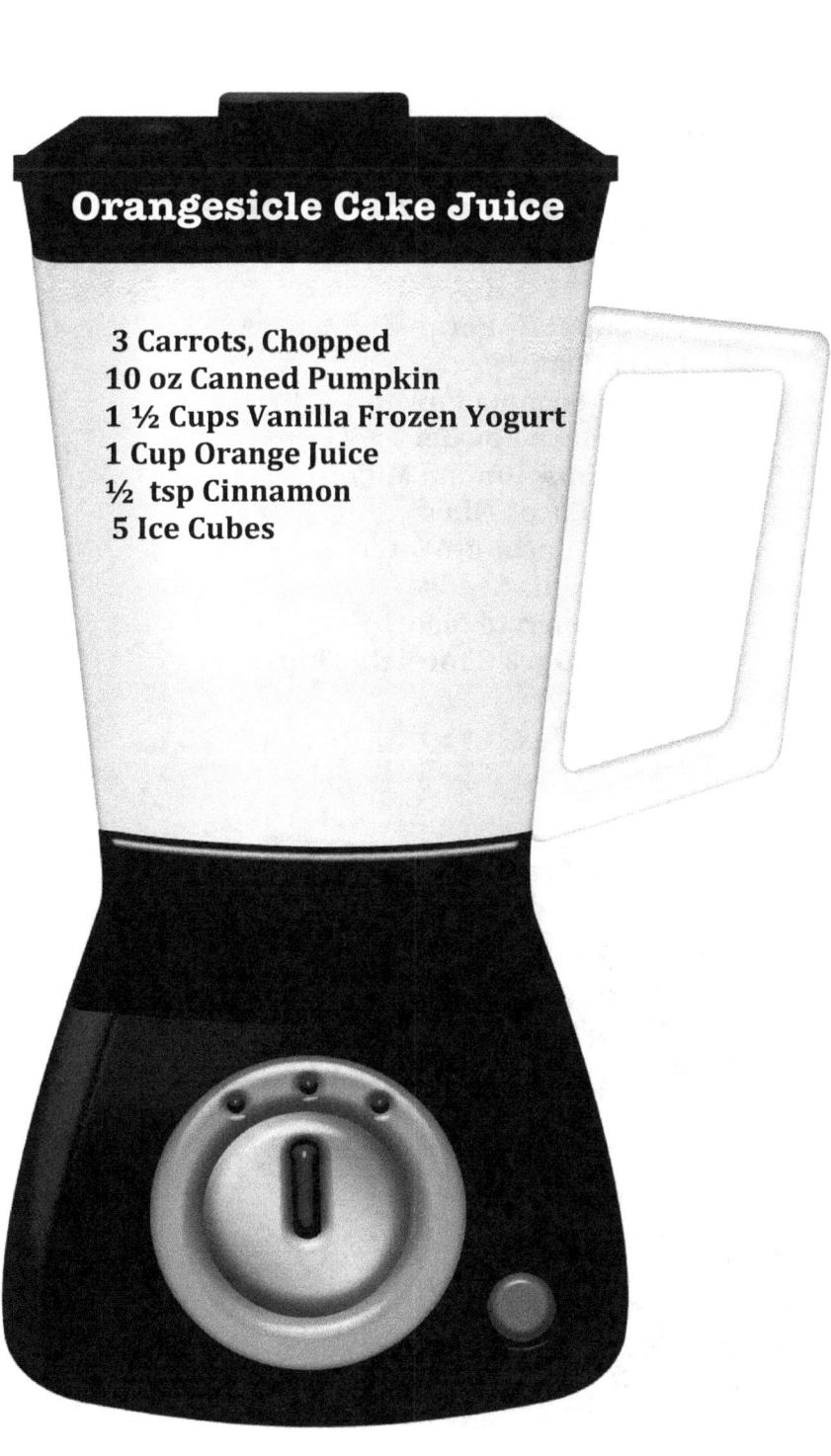

Orangesicle Cake Juice

3 Carrots, Chopped
10 oz Canned Pumpkin
1 ½ Cups Vanilla Frozen Yogurt
1 Cup Orange Juice
½ tsp Cinnamon
5 Ice Cubes

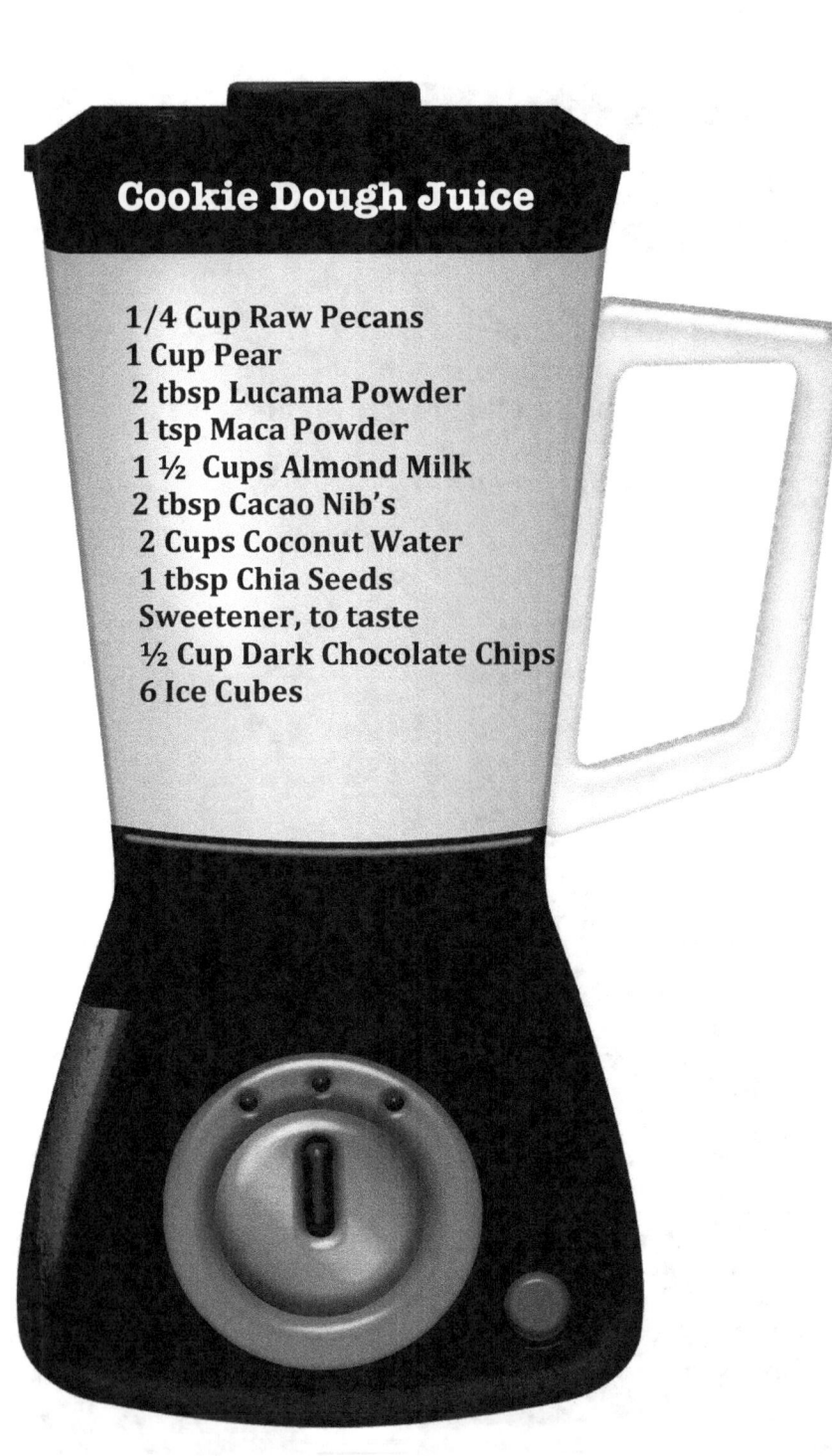

Cookie Dough Juice

1/4 Cup Raw Pecans
1 Cup Pear
2 tbsp Lucama Powder
1 tsp Maca Powder
1 ½ Cups Almond Milk
2 tbsp Cacao Nib's
2 Cups Coconut Water
1 tbsp Chia Seeds
Sweetener, to taste
½ Cup Dark Chocolate Chips
6 Ice Cubes

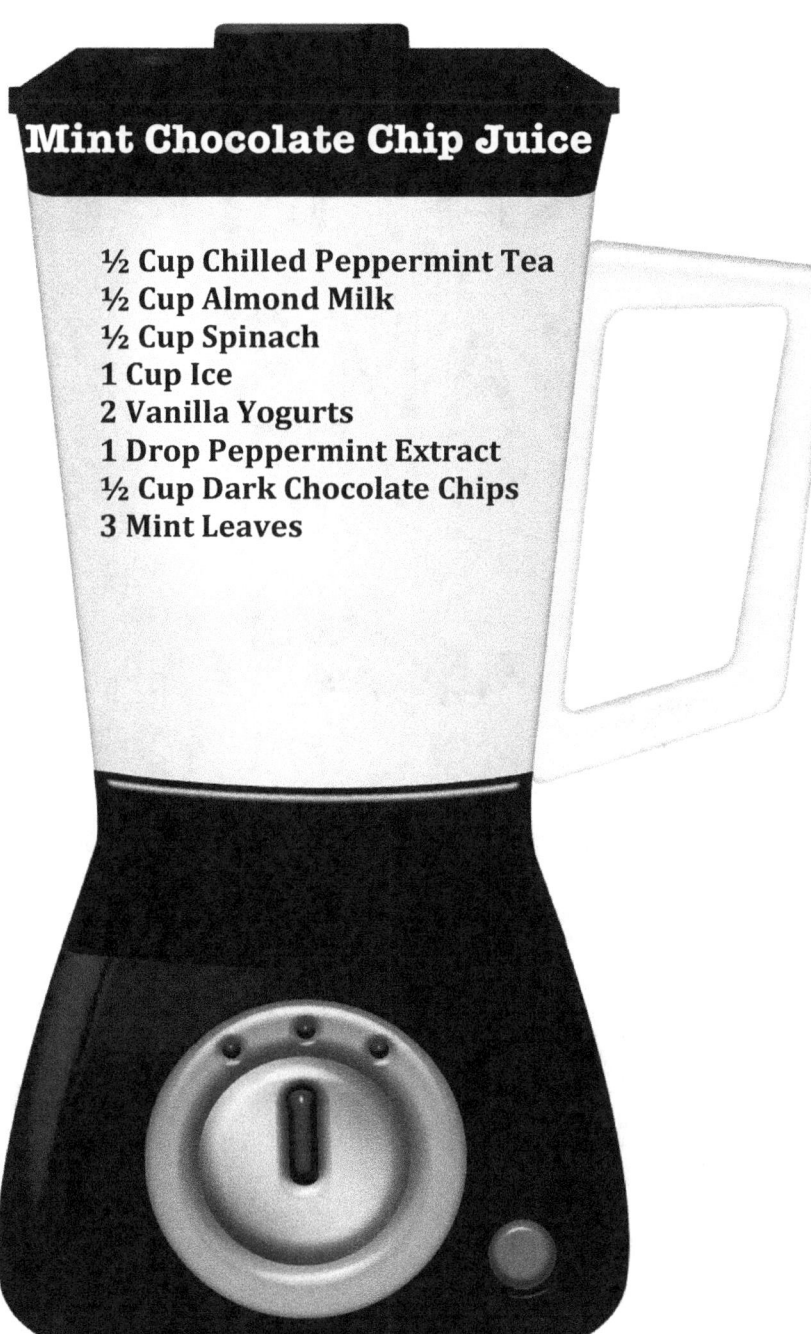

Mint Chocolate Chip Juice

½ Cup Chilled Peppermint Tea
½ Cup Almond Milk
½ Cup Spinach
1 Cup Ice
2 Vanilla Yogurts
1 Drop Peppermint Extract
½ Cup Dark Chocolate Chips
3 Mint Leaves

JUICY LIFE JAMS

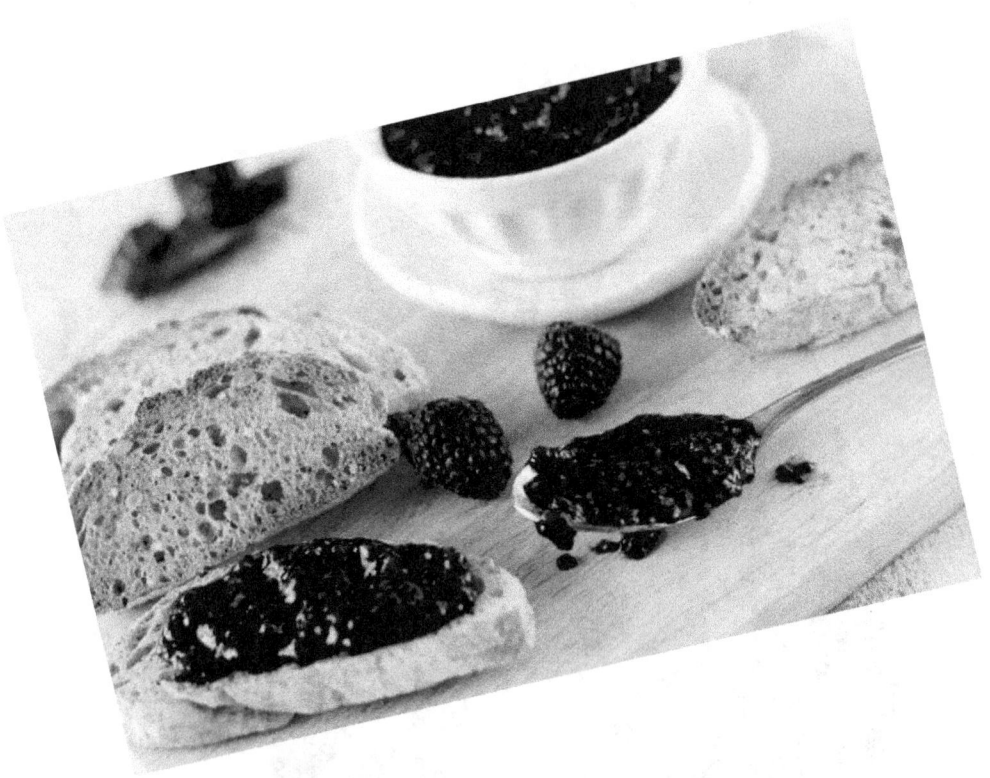

Berry Chia Jam

Ingredients

- 2 cups strawberries, de-stemmed and chopped in half
- 1 cup raspberries
- ¼ cup Agave
- 2 Tbsp Chia Seeds
- Water as needed
- 1 tablet Juicy Life Xtreme

Instructions

1. Place chopped strawberries, raspberries, chia seeds and agave into a blender. Blend on medium to high speed until preferred jam consistency is obtained. Add water 1 Tbsp at a time as needed to get things moving.
2. Pour contents of blender into a small saucepan and heat over medium heat until the jam begins to bubble. Reduce heat to low and simmer for 5-7 minutes, or until the jam starts to thicken.
3. Remove from heat and immediately pour into a mason jar. Allow to cool completely and then store in the fridge for up to one week.

Pineapple Chia Seeds

Ingredients

- 1 medium size pineapple
- 1 tablespoon tapioca pectin
- 1 tablespoon chia seeds
- ¼ teaspoon pure honey
- 1 tablet Juicy Life Xtreme

Instructions

1. Dice the pineapple and then puree in a blender with the tapioca pectin.
2. Pour the pineapple puree into a saucepan over medium heat. Cook and let the water evaporate. Stir continuously to prevent the jam from burning. Approximately 10 minutes.
3. Add chia seeds. Add stevia if you want extra sweetness.
4. Let the jam cool to room temperature and then store in a clean glass jar. It can be kept in refrigerator up to 10 days.

Banana Chia Seed

Ingredients

- 1/2 tbsp chia seeds
- 2 oz water
- 1/2 banana
- 1/2 tsp honey
- Cinnamon to taste
- 1 tablet Juicy Life Xtreme

Directions

1. Combine chia seeds with water in a bowl. Wisk vigorously for 30 seconds and set aside for 20 minutes until a gel is formed
2. Mash the bananas with a fork. Add the honey and cinnamon and mix together
3. Combine gel chia seeds with the mashed bananas
4. Can be served on top of toast as a "jam"

www.ingramcontent.com/pod-product-compliance
Lightning Source LLC
Chambersburg PA
CBHW072201280526
45788CB00002B/831